Fundamentals of Health at Work

T0186677

Fundamentals of Health at Work

The social dimensions

Carol Wilkinson

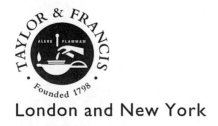

London and New York

First published 2001 by Taylor & Francis
11 New Fetter Lane, London EC4P 4EE

Simultaneously published in the USA and Canada
by Taylor & Francis
29 West 35th Street, New York, NY 10001-2299

Taylor & Francis is an imprint of the Taylor & Francis Group

© 2001 Carol Wilkinson

The publisher makes no representation, express or implied, with
regard to the accuracy of the information contained in this book and
cannot accept any legal responsibility or liability for any errors or
omissions that may be made.

Every effort has been made to ensure that the advice and information
in this book is true and accurate at the time of going to press.
However, neither the publisher nor the author can accept any legal
responsibility or liability for any errors or omissions that may be
made. In the case of drug administration, any medical procedure or
the use of technical equipment mentioned within this book, you are
strongly advised to consult the manufacturer's guidelines.

British Library Cataloguing in Publication Data
A catalogue record for this book is available from the British Library

Library of Congress Cataloguing in Publication Data
Wilkinson, Carol.
    Fundamentals of health at work : the social dimensions / Carol Wilkinson.
        p. cm.
    Includes bibliographical references and index.
    ISBN 0-419-24820-X -- ISBN 0-419-24830-7 (pbk.)
    1. Industrial hygiene--Great Britain. I. Title.

RC967 .W536 2000
613.6'2--dc21

                                                              00-04790

ISBN 0-419-24820-X (hbk)
ISBN 0-419-24830-7 (pbk)

Acknowledgement

This work began as a series of interconnected thoughts about the span of workplace health development, namely occupational medicine, health and safety regulations, workplace health promotion and occupational health. I had the opportunity of meeting and conversing with people who have encouraged me along the way, for which I am truly grateful. These include Richard Wynne, Andrew Tannahill, Erica Wimbush and Arun Midha. Also to Nancy Harding, Emeritus Professor Bill Williams, Barrie Long and David Rea for your faith in me as your student.

Special thanks, however, are reserved for Mick Carpenter. I hope we can continue to wrestle with these ideas and concepts on workplace health and illness.

Preface

This text is intended to be a re-assessment of issues of workplace health. There is particular emphasis on the neglected social context of workplaces and their impact on individuals.

In an attempt to wrestle with history and concepts of health and illness, there emerges a series of thoughts linking history, organisational development and health improvement, not by any means complete, and I apologise to those writers whom I have not included but the necessity to be selective, will hopefully become apparent in the reading.

The aim, is to engage the reader to begin to look beyond issues of legislation and safety and to recapture the essence of public health within our own time and to learn through history to develop and improve the health of people within our workplaces.

The text was partly written out of frustration concerning the limited reading material available on the phenomena of workplace health and illness in Britain. There is much on regulation and safety which exists in the main, not that there is a necessary detraction from these issues and ideas, for it is acknowledged that they bring a valuable contribution to our understanding of the field. However, the consideration of the social context of health and illness is neglected; its starting point, progression, its recovery and development is my aim.

This is merely the beginning of analysis and I hope others will in time join forces in picking up the threads.

My indebtedness is extended to the works of the late Bertil Gardell whom I discovered some eight years ago. This book does only small justice to aspects of his work. I hope the discoveries continue to develop and grow in time and that my readers do the same.

Carol Wilkinson

Contents

Acknowledgement   v
Preface   vi

1   The peculiarity of the workplace as harbinger of
    illness   1

2   The historical context   25

3   Regulatory developments, roles and functions   50

4   The work, the organisation and the individual   74

5   Theoretical perspectives of workplace health
    improvement   107

6   Workplace health promotion   143

    References   171
    Index   190

Chapter 1

The peculiarity of the workplace as a harbinger of illness

This chapter is intended to outline the issues that communicate illness within organisations. Using a framework of components of organisations as the starting point in analysis, a demonstration of how these components impact upon the individual and encourage illness is undertaken. What is considered to be the determinants of health at work will be expressed through interrogating aspects of the wellness–illness dichotomy.

Health at work

The notion of health within organisations is largely communicated as an add on to issues of safety, through health professionals emphasising a medical model of health, through literature such as what may be leaflets and posters communicating the how and the what, sometimes the why of health problems, as well as who may be affected. The facilities of the organisation also communicates the symbolism of health and illness. This may be immediately detected from the furnishings, reception, the language of the members of the organisation. How many times have you entered the front entrance of a council building or a hospital and witnessed the litter of used cigarette ends accompanied by signs clearly posted on the walls of the organisation stating 'No Smoking'?

Company manuals and policies marking out heavily worded legislation communicating *protection* and *responsibility* where the onus is usually upon the individual to keep the organisation safe, protected. It is the role of every employee to take responsibility for looking after the organisation. That is of course, the building, the environment in which they work.

This premise however, is rather simplistic. The organisation is made up of much more than the building and its environs. Responsibility within organisational terms rarely communicates well being, satisfaction, happiness, joy, physical fitness, emotional and spiritual well being. This is largely due to the fact that health within the organisation is invisible or at best connected to negative connotations like responsibility, discipline, accidents, sickness, absence and inability. One is not healthy, therefore one is unable to … perform, participate, act, fulfil the needs of the organisation.

A series of studies dating as far back as Ramazzini, through to Engels' ground breaking work in Manchester in the nineteenth century, the Marxian school, and the *Hazards at work* generations have brought confirmation of the phenomena of the sick organisation. Organisations are *illness* generating environments rather than ones where health is paramount. We need to explore why organisations are a harbingers of illness as opposed to wellness.

If we look at the components of the organisation as a framework, then observe their points of departure in analysis, we can begin to understand the peculiarities of the sick organisation. The sick organisation is pervasive, it is inherent within the organisation's structure and dynamic in that it develops a momentum of its own.

Components of the workplace

The individual – organisations are made up of their individual members. The individual is central to any form of organisational behaviour and a necessary part of any behavioural situation. This can range from acting in isolation or as part of a group. It will include individual actions in response to expectations of the organisation, or as a result of influences of the external environment. Where the needs of the individual and the demands of the organisation are incompatible, this can invariably result in frustration and conflict. The resulting tensions not only have an impact on the health of the organisation in the broader sense, but have health repercussions for the individual, their families and loved ones. It is supposed to be the task of management to provide a working environment which permits the satisfaction of individual needs as well as the attainment of organisational goals but this is not always the case as identified in many studies (including Stogdill and Coons 1957; Hersey and Blanchard 1988; Boumans and Landeweerd 1993). The working environment consists of and/or produces substances hazardous to the individual worker. Some are carcinogenic, others cause injuries in the case of asbestos, poly vinyl chloride and rapid paced machinery or technology (Davidson 1971; Dawson 1988; Pheasant 1991).

The group – groups exist in all organisations and are essential to their working and performance. The organisation is comprised of groups of people and almost everyone in an organisation will be a member of one or more groups. Informal groups arise from the social needs of people within the organisation. People in groups influence each other in many ways, and groups may develop their own hierarchies and leaders.

Group pressures can have a major influence over the behaviour and performance of individual members. An understanding of group structure and behaviour components combine with a knowledge of individual behaviour and adds a further dimension to organisational behaviour. Pressure to conform within groups can sometimes make for a sick organisation.

The issue of rights and ceremonials within an organisation heavily influences group behaviour (see Chapter 4). Rights of degradation can operate in the form of group process to strip individuals of powerful social identities and give them lesser ones. Powerful social statuses tend to be closely linked with individual identities. The rites of degradation dissect them and make them separate. Another person can inhabit and assume the powers of the now separated status of the target individual. The process involves rites of separation, discrediting rights and rites of removal (Fortes 1962; Garfinkel 1962).

Rites of separation begin when an organisation's members focus attention on persons to be degraded and publicly associate them with organisational problems and failures. The language of 'failure', 'belittling' and 'problem' is an important part of this process (Gephart 1978), thus discrediting the innocent individual. Rites of removal are depicted in subsequent managerial procedures to constructively dismiss the innocent individual. The underlying problems remain in this dysfunctional organisation where progress will never be made so long as the status quo continues to thrive. Any form of discriminatory behaviour within organisations can be associated with this process. Managers reinforce this process if they maintain cognitive dissonance.

Other examples of the dysfunctional organisation can be seen in frustrating and blocking the elevation of individuals up the organisational hierarchy (Trice and Roman 1971; Prange 1981).

The organisation – individuals and groups interact within the structure of the formal organisation. Structure is created by management to establish relationships between individuals and groups, to provide order and systems, and to direct the efforts of the organisation into goal seeking activities. It is through the formal structure that people carry out their organisational activities in order to achieve aims and objectives. Behaviour is affected by patterns of organisation structure, technology, styles of leadership and systems of management through which organisational processes are planned, directed and controlled. The focus of attention, therefore, is on the impact of organisation structure and design, and patterns of management, on the behaviour of people within the organisation.

Primary functions of organisations are intended to protect the well being of the organisation as opposed to the individual. Organisations are intended to be productive or economic. They are concerned with the creation of wealth, the manufacture of goods and the provision of services for the public. The role of maintenance is part of the process, for example, schools and churches, concerned with the socialisation of people to fulfil roles in other organisations and in society. They are intended to be adaptive to change. Research establishments for example, are concerned with the pursuit of knowledge and the development and testing of theory. As political negotiators, organisations operate to maximise influence, e.g. government departments assist in the adjudication of physical and human resources.

The primary functions of the organisation are often not compatible with the needs of the individual saving monetary terms and the supposed prevention of social isolation. The dichotomy between wellness and illness in the individual can also become integral to the operations of the organisation. The sick individual contributes to the sickness of the organisation's functions, capacity, workload, habits and cultures. Sickness can be pervasive, not merely in the physiological sense, but in an esoteric, linguistic, and psychological sense as well. Organisations can become enmeshed through their activities to breathe life and reinforce the sick organisation.

The environment – it affects the organisation through, for example, technological and scientific development, economic activity, social and cultural influences and governmental actions.

The way in which these components, the environment, organisation and groups impact on the individual affecting their health is an issue that requires greater consideration. It creates conflict, tension and inequalities within the workplace.

For some researchers health at work is seen as an environmental problem.

> ... in the largest number of references, work is conceived of as an environmental problem. It exposes individual workers to physical, chemical, and psychological agents that may make them sick or cause them to have accidents. The strategy of intervention derived from this understanding of work is to reduce the frequency of workers' exposure to pathological agents. While the enormous importance of this task should not be minimized, the theory and practice derived from that understanding of work reproduce the individual–environmental dichotomy, which seriously hinders the understanding of social relations that determine both the individual worker and the environment.
>
> Navarro 1982, p. 535

The capacity of social relations to impinge upon the individual, so reinforcing health problems is a concept that is underdeveloped and largely ignored. Emphasis rested on prevention and individual responsibility.

It is widely accepted that there is no one defining attribute to the motivation to work. There are however, a number of competing theories which bifurcate with the health–illness dichotomy. Early writers including Taylor (see Chapter 4) believed in economic needs of people. Workers would be motivated by obtaining the highest possible wages through working in the most efficient and productive way. Performance was limited by physiological fatigue. For Taylor, motivation was a comparatively simple issue – workers wanted higher wages. This rather crude explanation was superseded with an emphasis on social needs and the value and recognition of individuals within the work environment. For human relations theorists, defining the socio-technical systems approach is concerned with the interactions between both the psychological and social factors, and the needs and demands of people. Additional focus was later placed on the content and tasks in work providing meaning, and personal adjustment of the individual within the work situation.

Maslow's well trodden theory (see Chapter 4) of the hierarchy of needs provides an all encompassing perspective of the needs of individuals, from safety to self actualisation. The absence of any of these components provides an indication of the level of fulfilment of the individual. Applied to wellness–illness dichotomy, it provides a clear indication that the absence or frustration of any of these components is an indicator that the individual is likely to be predisposed to physical or psychosocial displacement.

It is inherently the case however, that people do not necessarily satisfy their needs in the work situation, and secondly, despite the fact that Maslow viewed satisfaction as the main motivational outcome of behaviour, job satisfaction does not necessarily lead to improved work performance.

More modern theories have focussed on feelings of individuals in the workplace. Adams' Equity Theory (1965) focuses on feelings and fair treatment in comparison to treatment of others. It is based on the notion of exchange. People, in this commodification thesis, evaluate their social relationships in the same way as buying or selling an item. People expect certain outcomes in exchange for certain contributions or inputs. Social relationships involve exchange in comparison with others. Feelings about equity of exchange are affected by the treatment they receive when compared with what happens to other people. Inequity in the workplace causes tension and unpleasantness. The presence of inequity therefore motivates the person to remove or to reduce the level of tension and perceived inequity. The magnitude of perceived inequity determines the level of tension. The level of tension determines the level of motivation. The motivation to gain can also create a host of very different relationships within the workplace where survival may well become a key feature. Forms of work organisations depicting flattened management structures, short term contracts, longer working hours relate very much to this stimulus–response type behaviour. It compounds the notion of the sick organisation.

Adams identified the consequences of inequity:

1   *changes to inputs* – this involves a reduction in the quality of work, leads to increased absenteeism, and withdrawal in the number of hours worked;

2   *changes to outcomes* – attempts are made to change working conditions, status, and recognition without change to inputs. This may be depicted in aggression and rebellion within the organisation;

3   *cognitive distortion of inputs and outcomes* – e.g. people can talk up their worth in terms of pay and qualifications. Compared to others this may be regardless of ability or experience.

4   *leaving the field* – request for transfer, absenteeism, resigning from the job, or from the organisation altogether. This is a drastic step but leaving the sick organisation may be a positive move for the individual.

5   *acting on others* – attempt to change the perception of others in relation to value and worth. An unfortunate step because it compounds inequity and presents a false impression of the recipients of such treatment. Inequity is a demotivator in organisations and can become cancerous and pervasive if not dealt with by managers within the organisation. This means observation, taking stock and making the appropriate changes where necessary, including the dissipation of bullying and other forms of harassment at work, a feature of the late twentieth century working environment.

6   *changing the object of comparison* – changing the reference group to whom comparison is made.

Where inequity flourishes in the workplace, then other forms of behaviour may come into play. This can be detrimental to the health of individuals. A phenomenon now being researched is that of bullying and harassment in the workplace. It is another means of acquiring power in the workplace. Bullies can achieve greater power from the selective associations they make. The study of organisations reveals that they create many unofficial roles for colleagues, including henchmen, spies, lackeys, sycophants or court jesters. To be in favour with an aggressor might be the best way to survive. The protection it offers might seem to free individuals from fear. The bully who has favourites creates conflicting rivalries in the working group. Those who are out of favour deeply resent those they feel receive special treatment; this can lead to a working environment with an in or an out group, fostering secretive behaviour, clans, cliques and clandestine operations. The favoured members feel at times untouchable; others feel pushed out. The risk to the favoured is that they can lose their status by falling out of favour. This culture is divisive, destructive and ultimately brings out the worst elements in individuals (Adams 1992). Quines' (1999) study demonstrated that staff at work who are bullied experienced lower levels of job satisfaction and higher levels of job induced stress, depression and anxiety.

The needs of individuals in the workplace

Generally speaking, individuals enter the workplace with a common set of expectations. When these expectations are no longer being met they find ways of achieving or leaving the organisation. However, on a more positive note, their needs often include:

1   *safe and hygienic working conditions* – to feel comfortable at work, free from disease and hazards, regardless of the type of work that is required within the confines of a job description;
2   *job security* – to be sure that they will continue to work in the same place and at the same job for as long as they are willing and able;
3   *challenging, satisfying work* – research over the years has demonstrated that a sense of fulfilment and well being can be achieved as long as the work enables the individual to make use of their talents and skills, as well as extend their capacity for development. Opportunities for personal and career development are also necessary. This implies finding meaning and joy in work (De Man 1929; Arendt 1958; Blauner 1964; Gardell 1982);
4   *policies and procedures* – knowing the formal/informal rules of the organisation. This provides structure for the individual to enable them to take the opportunity to operate within organisational and legal boundaries.

Concepts of health

The long established medical definition of health is one that is reliant on the absence of the condition which heralds some form of biological disruption of the body. Physiological functioning is reduced, therefore necessitating appropriate medical treatment in order to return the body to its original state of health. Health in this instance takes on the scientific notion of the absence of malfunction; the absence of disease.

This notion is clarified in that the medical definition of health implies there is no definition of health, but instead describes what is not disease. The arguments are well rehearsed in the works of Wolinksy (1988) in terms of objectivity, that is, measurable symptoms of illness, sole evaluation by the medical profession, power through judgement, underlining the physiological criteria and the residual nature of the definition. This links with the notion of two states, illness and wellness.

The World Health Organization (1946) originally identified health as the ' *... state of complete physical, mental and social well being and not merely the absence of disease and infirmity'*. This universally communicated definition by health professionals is not merely concerned with the absence of disease, it takes on a much broader perspective relating to the dimensions that affect daily living. The concept is not new. Foucault (1973) wrote that the notion of health as *'soundness of body, mind and spirit'* was a widespread concept until the end of the eighteenth century. The growth of the medical profession resulted in a change in understanding to health being seen as a state of biological normality which could be achieved through external intervention. Despite this lengthy history, the WHO's definition has been widely criticised as utopian and idealistic. It is an ideal that is immeasurable, it does not explain arrival at the state of well being or how it is achieved.

On a more positive note, it implied that individual and social action was necessary to achieve this state. In revising their definition, the WHO Working Group (1984) redefined health as '*the extent to which an individual or group is able on the one hand to realise aspirations and satisfy needs and on the other hand, to change or cope with the environment*'. Health is therefore seen as a resource for everyday life, not the objective of living: it is a positive concept emphasising social and personal resources as well as physical abilities.

Seedhouse's (1991) philosophical interpretation of health focuses on quality of life. He advocates a sense of striving to reach one's potential. Issues of health are not merely issues of medicine and disease. Health topics are inextricably linked to wider issues concerning how people can and ought to conduct their lives. Health for many people is the way in which a person is able to live regardless of physiological and psychological good fortune. Generally, he states that '*a person's health is equivalent to the state of the set of conditions which fulfil or enable a person to work to fulfil his or her realistic chosen and biological potentials*'. Working towards health is concerned with enabling people to achieve these potentials through laying the foundations and removing the barriers to achievement. This means that '*the goal of health for all*' is not the sole ownership of the medical profession.

Seedhouse's exposition does not go far enough in that he leaves us contemplating issues of early socialisation for health and encouraging cultural change. He underlined the fact that we should move beyond the '*barriers to achievement*'. However, if one starts from the premise of inequality in society where poverty, social class, 'race' and gender are problematic and structural, how can these barriers be broken down? What agencies within society can assist in this process?

Illness is a social construct (Parsons 1955; Wolinsky 1988; Gerhardt 1989). It is created within society by society. It is the product of social action, it produces its casualties and it is the product of social control. Inequality in society is a major cause of suffering in society. Illness arises through conflict that is raised wittingly or unwittingly within the society that individuals inhabit (Gerhardt 1989). In the same way, the expectations within organisations, that is, conformity to the organisation's principles, obedience to management regardless of punishments inflicted, loyalty to the organisation, merge and overlap to reinforce its dysfunction, reinforcing its illness behaviour and communicating itself within the individual.

Determinants of workplace health

The social determinants of workplace health is a position developed from the understanding that a health potential can be maximised through the recognition of individual and organisational needs. The wellness–illness dichotomy can be balanced if needs of both are balanced in terms of desires and expectations. At the same time emphasising the fact that specific requirements and situations need to be created in order for the individual to achieve optimal health and maintain an equilibrium as a result of work and enhance their quality of working life.

Research into organisational illness and well being as exhibited within the individual, has demonstrated that specific requirements are communicated in the illness forming behaviour and issues. It is with this knowledge that we can begin to realise a model determining workplace health. It is by no means complete and will continue to develop, grow and change as findings about organisational health becomes clearer. This is merely the beginning.

The social determinants of workplace health involve:

Control – lack of control over working systems and own work has been found to lead to the adverse result of stress, and a predisposition to cardiovascular problems (Gardell 1971; Frankenhauser 1988; Johnson 1991). The ability to influence corporate policy, negotiate aspects, terms, conditions of employment and immediate control of the work process is necessary for health and well being.

Skill – the process of deskilling and fragmentation of tasks at work has been linked to the issue of stress (Gardell 1966; Frankenhauser 1988).

Stimulation – an undernourished and underutilised brain at work leads to diminished performance and stimulation. Monotonous work reduces attentiveness and preparedness (Theorell 1987; Frankenhauser 1988).

Ability to Unwind and freedom of expression – this is regarded as a male privilege after work (Frankenhauser 1988; Hall 1991). The role of women and interaction between work and home needs to be considered. Emotion work in personal relationships at work are seen as a developing phenomenon (Meerbow and Page 1998).

Participation – people deal with poor work conditions, pressure and non participation by holding back human resources (Gardell 1987). Gardell saw participation as a political goal for dealing with work problems (Johnson et al. 1991).

Reduce emotion work – emotion work is bad for women in terms of the impact on health and modes of behaviour adopted (Frith and Kitzinger 1998). It leads them into acting in ways against their own best interests (Zadjow 1995). Performance of emotion labour over the long term produces feelings of ontological insecurity and sustains social divisions and inequalities of 'race' and gender at home and work (Freund 1998). Karasek and Theorell (1990) note that 'denial' of feelings has a distinct link to coronary heart disease.

Appropriate decision latitude – the most adverse reactions of physical strain i.e. fatigue, anxiety, depression and physical illness can occur when the psychological demands of the job are high and the workers decision latitude in the task is low (Karasek and Theorell 1990; Johnson 1991).

Interaction with others – this can have positive and negative effects physically and psychologically on the individual and so a balance needs to be struck in the workplace (Gardell 1971, 1977; Hochschild 1983; Fineman 1993). Passivity and social isolation has an impact on psychological and physiological functioning (Gardell 1977). Passivity crosses work and home life in terms of behaviour i.e. passivity at work, leads to passivity in home life, political life and is a feature of social alienation (Gardell 1982, 1987).

Support with work process/problems – the literature on social support indicates that human ties are an important factor in mental and physical health. There is still only limited information concerning social support in occupational settings (Johnson 1991). This predisposes men to cardiovascular disease (Marmot and Theorell 1988).

Ability to plan work tasks – role conflict, ambiguity, lack of control over-planning and work methods predisposes the individual to stress (Gardell 1980, 1982; Cooper and Williams 1994).

Equity and fairness – these issues can be socially resolved according to the research available through fostering democracy in the workplace (Gardell 1980, 1982). There has been a concerted attempt to break from the conventional view which cast the worker in the role of a relatively passive 'object' without voice or defence who could be acted upon by others. Workers are inherently subjects who not only respond to their environment but act formally and informally to change it.

Freedom from personal injury – injury prevention is a battle fought and won by the trade union movement. All employers have a statutory obligation to ensure the work environment is safe for employees which cannot be avoided, hence its inclusion in the determinants of a workplace health model (Table 1).

Work and health pre-1970s

Up to the early 1970s there was a theoretical focus on the degree of pressure or load placed on the individual worker by the demands of the production system.

Empirical investigations in this field have examined specific job design features such as machine-pacing, shift work, and piece rate payment systems, but have also considered broader issues involving the nature and structure of the work process itself. This model of workplace stress was analogous to the way an engineer would view the structural integrity of a bridge: how much load can it bear, and when does damage occur. However,

Table 1. Social Determinants of Workplace Health

- Exercising control over working systems and own work
- Demonstrating ability to use skills
- Stimulation through work
- Ability to unwind and freedom of expression
- Participation
- Reduce emotion labour
- Appropriate decision latitude
- Interaction with others
- Support with work problems/work process
- Ability to plan tasks
- Equity and fairness
- Freedom from personal injury

this relatively simplistic stimulus–response model had little success as yielded in explaining disease related to work exposure.

As a consequence, researchers began to examine aspects of the individual workers and their psychological environment that might serve to explain the differences observed in stress responses and disease rates within the working population. Two distinct approaches emerged. The first has focused primarily on the individual worker; generally, predispositions, attributes and skills. For the most part, these rested with cultural values and political inclinations of the time. Much of this research occurred in the United States. The other, from European researchers, particularly those in Sweden and Norway, tended to emphasise the structural characteristics of the work setting itself and had focused their attention on the resources available to individuals.

Assembly line manufacturing provided a rich source of data for illness at work. A great deal of work has been undertaken forging the link between conditions of a particular job and its relationship to physical and mental health. Kornhauser (1965) found the pace of work to be an issue. For example, that poor mental health was directly related to unpleasant work conditions, the necessity to work fast and to expend a lot of physical effort, and to excessive and inconvenient hours.

In addition to Kornhauser's findings, there grew increasing evidence (Marcson 1970; Shephard 1971) that physical health as well, is adversely affected by repetitive and dehumanising environments (e.g. paced assembly lines). Kritskis et al. (1968) for example, in a study of 150 men with angina pectoris in a population of over 4000 industrial workers in Berlin, reported that more of these workers came from work environments employing conveyor line systems than any other work technology. Studies into repetitive strain injuries during the 1980s and 1990s in factory and office environments has enhanced knowledge in this field (Westgaard and Aaras 1984, 1985; Grieco 1986; Willis 1986; Cleland 1987; Ferguson 1987; Fry 1988;

Ryan and Bampton 1988). RSI became a metaphor for alienation and the product of social iatrogenesis.

Work and health up to late 1980s

Studies of work and health can be grouped into two broad categories: those relating to physically dangerous occupational conditions to health; and those relating psychosocially stressful occupational conditions to health.

The majority of earlier work on stress and health has suffered from two limitations. First, they have failed to untangle the web of relationships between occupational conditions, work experience and subsequent health consequences. The usual approach had been to relate occupational conditions to health via the psychological distress certain occupational conditions are alleged to cause.

The limitations were recognised later, but it is with respect to consideration of social–psychological processes whereby occupational conditions can affect health (Schwalbe and Staples 1986). A second characteristic of research in this field tended towards an astructural bias. This was often depicted in work at the psychosocial level pre-dating visionaries such as Conrad and Johnson (Gardell 1966; Zaleznik et al. 1970; Coburn 1978, 1979; Garfield 1980; La Rocco et al. 1980; Navarro and Berman 1983).

By the late 1970s a small number of researchers had attempted to put the problem of work stress and health into a structural framework. The usual approach in these cases was to discuss the psychological distress produced by certain occupational conditions in terms of alienation, thus implying a historical materialist connection to a Marxist structural analysis of capitalism (see Navarro, Chapter 6). However, in these studies the Marxist framework is never fully developed. The analytical tool used for understanding relationships between work stress and health was not made entirely explicit. These studies therefore tended to lack social psychological rigour in proportion to their degree of structural emphasis. They have, however, subsequently provided the best guidance in continued critical sociological analysis of work stress and health (Schatzkin 1978; Coren 1980; Navarro 1982). It will be interesting to see if more sophisticated models of analysis are developed to interrogate this and other phenomena that contributes to the wellness–illness dichotomy in the workplace.

The rise in office and service occupations and the parallel decline in manufacturing industries, has brought concerns with work organisation, and stress has become more central to the field of occupational health. One indication of the growing importance of this area during the 1980s, is stress related disability claims where the most rapidly growing form of occupational illness within the Worker's Compensation system exists in the United States (Johnson and Hall 1988). This too has become an issue in the UK, particularly in reported illnesses amongst the medical profession as a result of work hours, workload and work stress (Mitchell et al. 1996; Quine 1999).

Levels of organisational analysis

Components of the organisation frequently included in analysis have also a direct link to the way in which illness develops. These very components impact upon the individual in different ways and can be communicated through issues relating to workload, frustration, powerlessness and demotivation. This has been demonstrated in many studies.

Workload

Role overload is when a person faces too many separate roles or too great a variety of expectations. The person is unable to meet satisfactorily all expectations and some must be neglected in order to satisfy others. This leads to a conflict of priority.

Role underload can arise when the prescribed role expectations fall short of the person's own perception of their role. The person may feel their role is not demanding enough and that they have the capacity to undertake a larger or more varied role, or an increased number of roles.

The issue of workload and its impact on the individual's predisposition to illness has been the subject of study for many years. Many of the main studies emerged during the late 1950s and continue to the present day. Some refinements have occurred with distinct focus shifting initially from disease oriented to more psychosocial conditions and their symbiotic relationship with the physical.

The main issue of the studies related to work and work process rather than combined home and work pressures (Garfield 1980). This latter phenomenon gained greater prominence in the late 1980s congruent with the increasing roles of women in the workplace, and the changes in work process and technology, particularly in the service sector.

Overwork and its subjective correlates also appear to be related to coronary disease. Over the generations we see the pattern repeating and extending amongst individuals and it has taken considerable time to communicate the messages of prevention amongst employers. Russek and Zohman (1958) reported that 91 out of 100 patients studied had experienced prolonged emotional stress associated with occupational demands prior to the onset of disease. Only 20 per cent of the control group had comparable experiences. Of the coronary group, 25 per cent had held two jobs and 46 per cent had worked 60 or more hours weekly. This holds implications for women who are predominantly part time workers. The pressures of raising a family and looking after the domestic environment is a situation that has not altered very much since Russek and Zohman's day. Occupational stress was reported to be a more important risk factor than diet, smoking, lack of exercise or family medical history (Hall 1991).

Sales (1969) provides additional research associating work overload and cardiovascular disease and several studies have linked working overtime with coronary heart disease (CHD). Relating work overload to coronary risk factors, French and Caplan (1972) indicated that:

> Our findings from several studies show that the various forms of work-load produce at least nine different kinds of psychological and physio-logical strain in the individual. Four of these (job dissatisfaction, elevated cholesterol, elevated heart rate and smoking) are risk factors in heart disease. It is reasonable to predict that reducing work overload will reduce heart disease.
>
> French and Caplan 1972, p. 44

From their preliminary findings in the above study, French and Caplan (1965, 1970, 1972) differentiated overload in terms of quantitative and qualitative overload. *Quantitative* referred to having too much to do while *qualitative* meant work that is too difficult to be dealt with at the pace required. Quantitative overload was strongly linked to cigarette smoking (an important risk factor or symptom of CHD). Persons with more phone calls, office visits and meetings per given unit of work time were found to smoke significantly more cigarettes than persons with fewer such engagements.

In earlier studies, French et al. (1965) looked at qualitative and quantitative work overload in a large university. They used questionnaires, interviews and medical examinations to obtain data on risk factors associated with CHD for 122 university administrators and professors. They found that one symptom of stress, low self esteem, was related to work overload but that this was different for two occupational groupings. Qualitative overload was not significantly linked to low self esteem among the administrators but was significantly correlated for the professors. The greater the 'quality' of work expected of the professor, the lower the self esteem. They also found that qualitative and quantitative overload were correlated to achievement orientation.

Quantitative overload is also seen as a potential source of occupational stress, as other studies (Quinn et al. 1971; Porter and Lawler 1965) indicate. A substantial investigation on quantitative workload was carried out by Margolis et al. (1974) on a representative national sample of 1496 employed persons, 16 years of age or older. They found that overload was significantly related to a number of symptoms or indicators of stress: escapist drinking, absenteeism, low motivation to work, lowered self esteem and a lack of goodwill on the part of employers to alter work pace and patterns to reduce illness and absenteeism.

Sickness is also equated with the social structure. As organisations often reflect the wider society, there is a tendency for repetition of the same factors for orientation to greater disease risk in the individual and malfunction within the organisation (Miller 1960; Terryberry 1968). Inequality, social exclusion, status and power are the same within the hierarchy of organisations.

Hierarchy, class and control

Power structures within the organisation create and reinforce specific patterns of behaviour and performance. This is reinforced through the hierarchy of the organisation and can be seen in behaviour, class and elements of control. Competition and striving when perceived to be 'logical' adaptations to organisations, tend to stratify workers into innumerable levels and rankings. The hierarchical division of labour and the myth of social mobility can promote the belief that work satisfaction, enhanced status and material comforts are attained by working hard enough, long enough and rapidly enough to achieve promotion within organisations.

Mettlin's (1976) research on type A behaviour (often considered to be competitive, aggressive, tense, striving) reveals the relationship of this coronary risk to the social organisation of work. Mettlin presents evidence that the type A pattern is *embedded in the social context of the modern occupational career*. He found type A characteristics were associated with rank in the occupational hierarchy, career mobility, perceived competitiveness of co-workers and employers' expectations that employees compete for promotions and salary increases, meet strict deadlines, do the most and best quality work possible and take work home to complete. In short, Mettlin's research suggests that type A behaviour is encouraged and reinforced by the work hierarchy.

In reality, social mobility for the majority of people, is rare and limited. It is considered according to some researchers, that meritocracy is a misnomer, especially where the issue of class plays a role within the organisation. Nepotism and favouritism as well as social networks compound this process. Some employees may find the glass ceiling weighing heavily upon them when these factors take over. People are 'tracked' from their earliest school days into occupational statuses corresponding to the class backgrounds of their families. Aronowitz notes that 'the hierarchy of occupations that results from a specific way of organising social labour gives credence to individual mobility aspirations even when mobility classes is foreclosed'. (Aronowitz 1974, p. 10).

There has been controversy connected to class position and stress not least in the work of Schwalbe and Staples (1986). They note that while supervisors, managers and the semi-autonomous employee frequently experiences stressful overload, the working classes typically experience debilitating underload. On the other hand, the old working class position of manufacturing industries during the 1970s and early 1980s associated with increased routinisation and therefore less stress. However, it was found that decreased control associated with working class position may increase stress under certain conditions. In this case, the psychological effects of class position were not theoretically unequivocal (Averill 1973; Lefcourt 1973; Cassell 1974; Frankenhauser and Gardell 1976; Gardell 1982; Fischer 1984).

Much of the experimental research concerning control up to the late 1970s had not made the distinction between control over and control within a situation. A simplified one dimensional control concept was frequently found in behaviouristic theories, where control was expressed in terms of mutual conditioning. Such theories neglected the asymmetry in situations characterised by inequality in power. In such situations the more powerful actor also controlled the rules of the situation. The individual, using various forms of psychological power games, created the structure of the situation and the rules, and also had the power to change the situation and the rules. For working life research that aims to contribute to better jobs, this distinction is necessary. Many industrial and office jobs during this period were one sided and deskilled employees to the extent that a strategy for job changes was communicated by researchers such as Lacey (1979) to increase a sense of well being amongst employees at all levels of the organisation.

One concept that has been extensively studied in this research and has a close relationship to social class is *decision latitude*, which was introduced by Karasek (1976). The first measure of decision latitude was constructed on the basis of the American Quality of Employment Surveys. A series of factor analyses were performed which indicated that decision latitude had two components: skill discretion and authority over decisions. These closely related statistically, and in most studies the two dimensions have been added to one another. It could be assumed, on theoretical grounds, that skill discretion may be a more basic dimension than authority over decisions. When workers have the possibility to learn new skills they can also master unpredicted future situations in a much better way, and since they feel more secure in their role they may be ready and able to make more and more decisions on their own, which of course, means increasing decision latitude. Fellow workers and supervisors will also know that such workers can make more decisions and will therefore allow them to do so. Almost by definition, both skill discretion and authority over decisions decrease with descending social class (Karasek 1988).

The concept of *control of destiny* has been applied to investigations into the working lives of civil servants. It was found that the lower people are in the socio-economic status hierarchy, the less chance they have to do what they need to do to live as they wish to live and the less chance they have to command the events that affect their lives. They have least influence and power within the social world and in the organisation. The lower down people are in the structure, the fewer opportunities and options they have for controlling their lives. This disposition includes not only structural limitations because of people's position in the social structure but also, the fewer resources and less training that people have to take advantage of opportunities and options, the less they are able to develop and flourish.

In the Whitehall Study of British Civil Servants, Marmot and Theorell (1988) took the opportunity to investigate the links between social position and rates of disease distribution. They found that there was a steep inverse association between grade (level) of employment and morality from CHD and a range of other causes. This gradient was steeper than demonstrated on a national basis when mortality was compared across the Registrar-General's scale of social class by occupation.

Frustration at work and powerlessness

Frustration and powerlessness are inherently connected to the structure of the organisation. If a person's motivational driving force is blocked before reaching a desired goal, there are two possible sets of outcomes: *constructive behaviour* or *frustration*.

Constructive behaviour is a positive reaction to the blockage of a desired goal and can take two main forms, either problem solving or restructuring. Problem solving is the removal of the barrier; for example repairing a damaged machine, or by-passing an unco-operative supervisor. Restructuring, or compromise, is the substitution of an alternative goal: although such a goal may be of a lower order, for example, taking a part time job.

Frustration is a negative response to the blockage of a desired goal and results in a defensive form of behaviour. There are many possible reactions to frustration caused by the failure to achieve a desired goal. These can be summarised as aggression, regression, fixation and withdrawal.

Wolf (1969) associates the 'Sisyphus Complex', characterised by relentless, ungratifying striving and prolonged, unresolved frustrations, with myocardial infarction and sudden death. This pattern includes dissatisfaction in work and leisure. Employers or those who engage in group activity to frustrate an employee are in effect attempting to disturb the equilibrium of their daily lives at work and home. In effect they are slowly killing that individual. Research on coronary-prone type A behaviour suggests that type A individuals are engaged in a relatively chronic struggle to obtain an unlimited number of poorly defined things from their environment in the shortest period of time, and if necessary, against the opposing efforts of other things or persons in the same environment. Highly committed to their treadmill existence, type As may stringently repress their often considerable frustration, hostility and insecurity. Thus subjective aspects of alienation – experiences of dissatisfaction and frustration – appear to be psychological factors in coronary heart disease.

There is a high requirement for fulfilment through work and achievement. Researchers found that the lack of promotional prospects and time to achieve promotion was significantly related to psychiatric illness (Arthur and Gunderson 1965).The internally motivated individual can find powerlessness within an organisation as a major contributory factor to ill health. Taylor (1969) suggests that *career development stress* is rooted in Freudian theory which suggests that work has value solely as a utility for individualistic motives of 'getting on in the world' and the desires of fame and success. This was confirmed by Kleiner and Parker (1963), who proposed a general theory which linked frustrated work aspirations to mental disorder. This was depicted in their results, from a later and larger study with urban Negroes (Parker and Kleiner 1966) which supported their hypotheses.

Another set of studies demonstrated that when the exercise of discretion in work is curtailed by spatial, temporal or technical restrictions built into the *work process*, the individual's ability to develop active relations during his spare time will diminish also. Persons whose jobs entail serious constraints with respect to autonomy and social interaction at work take far less part in organised and goal oriented activities outside work that require planning and co-operation with others (Gardell 1966; Meissner 1971; Westlander 1976). Thus social isolation and reduced sense of community can become a contributory factor. Although the research does not account for age, this is more likely to affect those who are settled into a relationship with commitments and family responsibilities where social mobility once the frustration becomes imminent is simply not an option.

Job dissatisfaction

The theoretical foundation for the idea of satisfaction or dissatisfaction is based on humanistic psychology and the idea that the individual enters the world with a reasonably well structured system of needs. Maslow developed the most widely applied example of this theory (see Chapter 4). Satisfaction is thought to indicate need fulfilment, while dissatisfaction indicates the reverse.

The lack of need fulfilment is thought to lead, through various processes, to the development of certain types of disease, at least if the dissatisfaction is prolonged (Gustavsen 1988).

This is a case in point. While numerous studies associate job dissatisfaction with coronary disease, Palmore's 15 year prospective study of longevity reports:

When the six strongest independent variables (work satisfaction, happiness rating, physical functioning, tobacco use, performance IQ and leisure activity) are combined in a step-wise multiple regression, work satisfaction is the best all over predictor of the LQ (Longevity Quotient) and explains about half of the final cumulative variance explained. This work satisfaction score represents a person's reaction to his general usefulness and ability to perform a meaningful social role.

Palmore 1969, p. 249

This is developed further in studies by Theorell and Rahe (1972), Lilijefors and Rahe (1970) and Sales and House (1971) and the findings taken forward into the works of contributors of the Scandinavian school of workplace health particularly during the 1970s to early 1990s (see Chapters 6 and 7).

Job dissatisfaction and stress have, from a scientific viewpoint, a number of elements in common. Firstly, they are both based on an idea that it is possible to define humans in terms of a number of 'internal states' that can be made subject to measurement. Secondly, they approach the human environment in the same way: as another set of measurable states. Thirdly, these states of people and environment can be linked to each other by cause and effect relationships or at least correlations, which are sufficiently strong to form the basis for ameliorative action; and finally, the relationship between the person and work can – and should – be split up into a series of two factor cause and effect relationships, e.g. between noise and its effect between organisation of work and its effect upon the individual (1980).

Research on monotonous work has emphasised several aspects of monotony. One line of research has focused on monotonous work as related to work motivation, alienation, job satisfaction, general life satisfaction, job socialisation and life outside work. Within a traditional ergonomic framework, psychological analyses have concentrated on information processing and means to optimise individual work output, while medical research has emphasised the development of musculo-skeletal disorders as a result of repetitive body movements. Finally, monotonous work has been subject to research concerning psychological stressors that have traditionally been acknowledged in the workplace, for instance, high physical and mental demands, excessive work, and time pressure. Further research has identified psychosocial stressors of a different kind. When factors such as understimulation, underutilisation of skills, few opportunities to learn new things on the job, and lack of autonomy and social support were brought into focus, they were also found to be associated with perceived strain, heightened sympathetic nervous system activity and morbidity (Conrad 1960; Kohn and Schooler 1983; Volpert 1986; Hagberg 1987).

Working hours

The most obvious aspect of work organisation that affects recovery time and leisure activities is shift work and other forms of irregular working hours. Disturbances in the diurnal rhythms of important bodily functions like temperature, heart rate and various hormones that regulate the activity level of the brain are found especially among rotating shift workers in various occupations. This may explain the sleeping problems and gastrointestinal disturbances found among these workers. Workers both on continuous and two shift systems have been found to participate less than daytime workers in political, trade union, social and cultural activities. On the basis of this research, The Swedish Metal Workers Union has asked for reduced working hours for two shift workers (Akerstedt 1979; Magnusson and Nilsson 1979).

This phenomena can also be linked to the role of working women who predominantly have less time for winding down and relaxing at home after a day's work especially when family and domestic chores call for greater attention than the self (see Chapter 6).

The working hours, length of work time and the correlation between illness is not new. Breslow and Buell (1960) have also reported findings which support a relationship between hours of work and death from coronary disease. In an investigation of mortality rates of men in California, they observed that workers in light industry under the age of 45, who are on the job more than 48 hours per week, have twice the risk of death from CHD compared with similar workers working 40 hours or less per week.

However, there continues to be overwhelming and disturbing evidence to link sickness and working hours. Although work hours have reduced for some since the 1960s, those in the service sector still experience lengthy working hours. Increasing consumer demand and knowledge about services has predominantly contributed to increased work time. Additionally, those leaving the service such as the professions of medicine, nursing and secondary education during the late 1990s, are not being replaced quickly enough, creating a domino effect in terms of workload and provision.

The UK's working week is unique compared to the average working week in the European Union. Along with the Netherlands and Denmark, the UK also has a high proportion of employees working shorter hours, reflecting in large part, the higher participation rate of women in the workforce. About half (some 48.5 per cent) of the population do some weekend work, 13.2 per cent work shifts and 1.9 per cent do night work. Some 66 per cent of Bangladeshi men and 60.1 per cent of Chinese are currently employed in the UK's catering industry. The industry is characterised by poor pay, long hours, shift working and insecurity of tenure. The rapidly changing needs of the market and the consumer often leaves this group as casualties of market forces.

There is a slightly different emphasis in the nursing and medical professions which predispose them to health problems. Several studies of junior doctors have uncovered high levels of depression, stress and burnout (Firth-Cozens 1987, 1995; Humphris et al. 1994). The same is true amongst hospital consultants and general practitioners (Porter et al. 1985; Winefield and Anstey 1991; Sutherland and Cooper 1992; Caplan 1994; Kirwan and Armstrong 1995; McKevitt et al. 1996). A continuous change in the National Health Service (NHS) in the drive towards efficiency and effectiveness, as well as longer working hours, have contributed to this process (Chambers and Belcher 1992; McKevitt et al. 1996).

For nurses, short term absence is a particular problem. There is growing evidence relating to absenteeism, stress and job dissatisfaction (Seccombe and Ball 1992; Seccombe and Buchan 1993). Trilio (1989) and Simpson (1990) recognise that nurses' working environments are places where behaviours are controlled and strictly guided along narrow lines. Nurses' clinical autonomy is limited, individual growth is discouraged and 'deviants' punished. Role ambiguity, mental and physical overload, as well as working hours have resulted in ill health.

Roles and relationships

A 'role' is the expected pattern of behaviours associated with members occupying a particular position within the structure of the organisation. It also describes how a person perceives the situation (Mullins 1994). Role incompatibility arises when a person faces a situation in which contradictory expectations create inconsistency. Compliance with one set of expectations makes it difficult or impossible to comply with other expectations. The two role expectations are in conflict.

Role ambiguity occurs when there is lack of clarity as to the precise requirements of the role and the person is unsure what to do. The person's own perception of their role may differ from the expectations of others. This implies that insufficient information is available for the adequate performance of the role.

Much of the research on role ambiguity and role conflict was launched following the seminal investigations of the Survey Research Center of the University of Michigan which were reported in the classic book *Organisational Stress: Studies in Role Conflict and Ambiguity* (Kahn et al. 1964). Role ambiguity exists when an individual has inadequate information about his work role, that is, where there is a lack of clarity about the work objectives associated with the role, about work colleagues' expectations of the work role and about the scope and responsibilities of the job.

Kahn et al. (1964) found that men who suffered more role conflict had lower job satisfaction and higher job related tension. It is interesting to note that they also found that the greater the power or authority of the people 'sending' the conflicting role messages, the more job dissatisfaction produced by role conflict. This was related to physiological strain as well. The Goddard study (French and Caplan 1970) illustrates this. They telemetered and recorded the heart rate of 22 men for a 2 hour period while they were at work in their offices. They found that the mean heart rate for an individual was strongly related to his report of role conflict.

A larger and medically more sophisticated study by Shirom et al. (1973) found similar results. They collected data on 762 male kibbutz members aged 30 and above, drawn from 13 kibbutzim throughout Israel. They examined the relationships between CHD (myocardial infarction, angina pectoris and insufficiency), abnormal electrocardiograph readings, CHD risk factors (systolic blood pressure, pulse rate, serum cholesterol levels, etc.) and potential sources of occupational stress (work overload, role ambiguity, role conflict, lack of physical activity). Their data were broken down by occupational groups: agricultural workers, factory groups, craftsmen, and white collar workers. It was found that there was a significant relationship between role conflict and CHD (specifically, abnormal electrocardiographic readings), but for the white collar workers only.

The job itself can produce conflicting findings in terms of predisposition to sickness at work. There are a number of studies (up to the mid-1960s) which related occupational level to CHD and MIH, of which Marks (1967) provides an excellent review. The majority of these studies supported the proposition that risk of CHD rises with occupational level (Ryle and Russell 1949; Breslow and Buell 1960; Syme et al. 1964; Wardell et al. 1964; McDonough et al. 1965). Substantial national analyses of both British and American mortality data lend support to these studies.

Not all researchers, however, were in agreement. Pell and D'Alonzo (1958) in a highly self consistent longitudinal study of Dupont employees found that incidence of myocardial infarction was inversely related to salary roll level. Stamler et al. (1960) and Bainton and Peterson (1963) also provided contradictory results. A further group of researchers compounded the confusion by finding no relationship between CHD and occupation; Berkson (1960) for blue versus white collar Negroes, Spain (1960) for Jewish salesmen versus other occupational groupings and Paul (1963) for different job levels at the Western Electric Co. As we have seen already, however, substantial studies since that time have overwhelmingly proven the case between CHD risk and different types of occupation and stress.

Some behavioural scientists (Argyris 1964; Cooper 1973) have suggested that good relationships between members of a work group are a central factor in individual and organisational health. This has also developed in the field of organisational culture, particularly in the works of Schein (1981, 1982, 1983, 1985). French and Caplan (1973) define poor relations as those which include low trust, low supportiveness, and low interest in listening to and trying to deal with problems that confront the organisational member.

The most notable early studies in this field are by Kahn et al. (1964), French and Caplan (1970) and Buck (1972). Both the Kahn et al. and French and Caplan studies came to roughly the same conclusion: that mistrust of persons one worked with was positively related to high role ambiguity, which led to inadequate communications between people and to psychological strain in the form of low job satisfaction and to feelings of job related threat to one's well being.

Activity level is usually regarded as a dimension which is important for the integration of people in the larger society, family life and cultural participation. In the context of stress research, activity level may also be seen as part of the worker's resources necessary to rely on in order to deal effectively with health and safety issues at the workplace. The lack of a social network and social isolation demonstrates an increase in physiological predisposition to ill health. A study by Knox et al. (1985) demonstrated that young men in Sweden aged 28 years working in non-learning occupations were more likely to have high levels of plasma adrenaline at rest and high systolic blood pressure at rest. This was the case regardless of the evidence of a job classified as boring. Conversely, it must also be emphasised that individual motivations to overwork can be induced and reinforced by alienating social structures, invariably through manipulated job settings, the hierarchical division of labour and contingent cultural patterns.

Technology

Technology increases the potential for illness at work. New technologies have caused many ill effects at the workplace. Poorly designed technology work stations have caused carpal tunnel and other ergonomic problems. The design of industrial and office systems have increased the potential for work load factors and placing workers in greater social isolation while being electronically monitored. Furthermore, computer-aided production has led to more continuous operation, especially in manufacturing but also in services. This has meant more shift work, another demonstrable source of stress and a contributor to illness at work (ILO 1981, 1983; Brown 1985).

The application of micro electronics has been a major source of change at the workplace since the late 1970s. The early *Detroit automation,* important during the 1950s and 1960s, was largely limited to mass production and assembly manufacturing production. In contrast, the silicon chip made the new microelectronic technology highly flexible and inexpensive; hence it has been applied in manufacturing and service sectors throughout industry. Illnesses associated with computer technology have become a feature of late twentieth century occupational medicine. NIOSH estimated that 15–20 per cent of the workforce is at risk of musculo-skeletal problems. Ergonomic problems also exist in the areas of manufacturing and increasingly in automated offices where video display terminals (VDTs) are in use (Bradley

1983; Tabor 1983; Slutzker 1985). The epidemic of repetitive injuries during the mid-1980s in Australia became a case in point. The majority of workers affected included keyboard operators, and those in the metal manufacturing industries. In Britain there are currently 20,000 people receiving treatment for some form of repetitive strain injury (HSE 1999).

Conclusion

Sickness is within and pervasive throughout the entire organisation. Sickness is structural and dynamic. It is not simply a biological process triggered by chemicals, or the fabric of the organisation. It is stimulated and perpetuated by its people through group process, action and behaviours at every level of the organisation. We need to move from the condition of illness to wellness within organisations. The process of achieving health is complex in light of the complexity of the progress towards illness. The remainder of this text is intended to develop further thoughts about the organisation, the historical and social processes that compound illness at work and home. The final chapter is intended to proceed to further developments in health and assess the ideas about the healthy organisation and the influence of health promotion. Some of the notions will be familiar, others not. The aim is to drive the process of thinking about health improvement at work with due consideration to the social context.

Chapter 2

The historical context

Workplace health in Europe is beginning a new era. At the end of the twentieth century, the issue of stress has become a major concern inside and out of the workplace. The now recognised total workload that people undertake in the private and public domain has resulted from the pressures of work, increased insecurity, short term contracts, commuting, restricted childcare provision and the recognition of unemployment of a partner have all formed part of the circle in which health figures greatly. However, progress has been made in legislation to protect both employee and employer, and the issue of health promotion at work is becoming a common feature, supported by governments and health professionals alike. Occupational health services too, are on the verge of change as there is now enough evidence to indicate activities in such a service coming closer to the health promoting philosophy.

Although the world has changed and services, ideas, philosophies in health continue to be observed and debated, arriving at this stage in workplace health development has been a tough one. The end of the twentieth century sees a greater convergence between occupational health and health promotion. This has not always been the case. Both have their own evolutionary and fragmented histories. This chapter intends to outline some of the issues that have marked out the combined work and health phenomenon.

Some of the earliest developments in the world of workplace health emerged from the mining industry. Observations of the diseases of miners were undertaken by Agricola (1494–1555) and Paracelsus (1493–1541). The expansion of mining during the middle ages from a feudal enterprise to becoming a skilled occupation, made strides in the contribution to the emancipation of the miner, particularly in Central Europe. As mining became more ambitious, the worse the conditions of work became, subsequently having an effect on the health of its workforce.

Agricola was appointed as physician in the town of Joachimstal in 1521. It was a flourishing metal mining centre where he witnessed some of the conditions that afflicted men who participated in such work. In *De Re Metallica* (Agricola 1556), published after his death, a record was kept outlining prevalence and cause of death. Similar studies were undertaken by Paracelsus of the Austrian experience, Ellenborg (c.1435–1499) in gold mining, mercury and the prevention of lead poisoning.

Bernardo Ramazzini (1633–1714)

The most substantial work to be developed in occupational diseases prior to the industrial revolution in Europe can be credited to Bernardo Ramazzini. Ramazzini drew particular attention to conditions such as stone masons and miners phthisis (now known as pneumoconiosis) and the eye problems associated with the work of gilding and printing. In 1700, he published *De Morbis Artificum Diatriba* based on his observations of workers in a series of occupations. He was influenced by the works of others in this field and reflected upon the impact for care and treatment of the worker in general.[1] In fact, Ramazzini was the first to make recommendations for physicians to take note of the occupation and social situation of working men and women when making a formal diagnosis. This opened up an entirely new branch of medical study, which later became established in the twentieth century although there were many difficulties in developing the academic discipline.

Of bricklayers he wrote:

> Workers of this sort are mostly drawn from the peasant class; so, when they are attacked by fever they betake themselves to their huts and leave the affair entirely to nature; or else they are carried off to hospitals and they are treated, like everybody else, with usual remedies, purging and venesection. For doctors know nothing of the mode of life these workers who are exhausted and prostrated by unceasing toil
> ...
>
> Ramazzini 1700, p. 449

The emphasis on social class came through identifying the relations between the health status of a given population within their living conditions and the connected work undertaken by this group.

The industrial revolution had developed in Europe. Closer to home, in Britain, the land enclosures and movement of people from the countryside to cities in pursuit of work meant entrepreneurs and factory owners erected homes for workers nearby. They were often poorly heated and ventilated. This was a time also of poor sanitation and cramped conditions, long work-

---

[1] Influence came from the works of Marsilio Ficino (c.1497) who wrote about the diseases of scholars; Grataroli (1555) and Horst (1615) on the health of scholars; Glauber (1657) on the health of seafarers; Porizio (1685) and Screta (1687) on soldiers diseases at camps, e.g. camp fevers.

ing hours and an industry that took advantage of child labour. Poor home and work conditions were part of the same equation for the majority of the working population.

There were a series of contributors who were able to make accounts and alter the effects of industrialisation on worker health. Many of these are associated with the nineteenth century – a period of reform in terms of working conditions, public health activity and trade unionism.

Although public health was inherent in the development of health improvement in society in general, there were specific contributions to workplace health advancement in the period. The following section outlines the main contributions of selected reformers of the period.

Contributions of selected reformers of the period

Thomas Percival (1740–1804)

Percival was a Manchester physician who was asked by the people of Ratcliffe in Lancashire to investigate an epidemic of typhus. It was during this time that he also made an investigation into the conditions and hours of employment of young workers. His report found favour with Peel. It contributed to the first Factory Bill, which became known as The Health and Morals of Apprentices Act 1802. The Act limited the number of hours of work per day to 12. Accommodation was made for religious and secular education and demanded the ventilation and lime-washing of workrooms. This legislation was followed by the Ten Hour Act of 1847 which restricted the hours of work for women and young persons to 58 hours per week.

Robert Owen (1771–1858)

Owen was a social reformer, born in Newtown, Powys Wales. He became manager and part owner of the New Lanark cotton mills, Lanarkshire, where he set up a social welfare programme, and established a 'model community'. His socialistic theories were put to the test in other experimental communities, such as at Orbiston, near Glasgow, and New Harmony in Indiana, but all were unsuccessful. He was later active in the trade union movement, and in 1852 became a spiritualist.

In New Lanark, Owen focused on issues relating to education and the improvement of the work environment. He refused to employ any young persons under the age of 10 and also shortened hours of work for the workforce generally. Owen also ensured that provisions were made for both adult and child education and made adjustments to the work environment which increased its equability. His mills, at least, were financially successful.

Owen persuaded Sir Robert Peel to introduce legislation to protect young persons in all types of textile mills, to prohibit the employment for those under 10 years and limit the working hours of minors to 10 hours per day. The Bill was passed in the House of Commons in 1819.

Charles Turner Thackrah (1795–1833)

Thackrah, a physician from Leeds, was the first to publish any British work on occupational medicine. His work entitled *The Effects of the Principal and Professions and of Civic States and Habits of Living on Health and Longevity* published in 1832.

Anthony Ashley Cooper, Lord Shaftesbury (1801–1885)

Shaftesbury was an evangelist and aristocrat who spent a considerable part of his life attempting to relieve the conditions of the destitute and deprived in Victorian England. As a member of parliament, he advocated the promotion of legislation which reduced the hours and improved conditions of work, particularly for women and young children. Many of his proposed reforms were bitterly opposed by entrepreneurs, but his power and influence did much to relieve the oppressive conditions created by the industrial revolution. He is credited with initiating the Factories Act 1833, whose impetus is documented in the Royal Commission's Report of the same year: ' ... the long working hours and bad conditions of labour to which children were subjected, damaged their physique, deprived them of education, and in some cases caused incurable disease and deformity.' (Battiscombe 1974, p. 90). As a result of these findings, the Ten Hours Act was passed forbidding children and young persons to work more than 10 hours per day.

Shaftesbury also contributed to the passing of the Miners Act in 1842. This feat was described as 'the most striking of Ashley's personal achievements' (Battiscombe 1974, p. 148). Shaftesbury, along with Southwood-Smith, presented drawings at the First Report of the Commissioners of Mines in 1842 which depicted some of the horrors of the mining industry and the work undertaken by children. It was this depiction which led to the passing of the Act. His involvement also spanned the Board of Health between 1848 and 1854.

Edward Headlam Greenhow (1814–1888)

Greenhow is credited with being one of the most outstanding epidemiologists of his generation. He made use of unpublished findings of the General Register Office to examine occupational mortality in more detail. He compared crude death rates from pulmonary disease in the lead mining towns of Alston and Reith in the North of England, with those of nearby Haltwhistle which had no lead mines.

Greenhow concluded that much of the increased mortality from pulmonary disease in England and Wales was due to the inhalation of dust and fumes arising from the work environment. His work influenced the Royal Commission to the extent that Factory Inspectors were given powers under the Factory Acts of 1864 and 1867 to enforce occupiers to control dust by fans or other mechanical means.

John Thomas Aldridge (1822–1899)

Aldridge was a physician in the pottery district of North Staffordshire, who devoted himself to the study of the diseases of potters. Aldridge spent much of his early career compiling statistics of those people working in the potteries which gravely reflected on the humanity of the manufacturers. He was instrumental in influencing the appointment of factory surgeons for earthenware and china manufacturers. Unfortunately, he never found favour with his medical colleagues.

Two hundred years of occupational safety and health legislation: a brief review

The Industrial Revolution in Britain saw many consequences for ordinary working people in terms of their livelihood, family relationships and gender divisions in and outside work. For the most part, this period of expansion and development from around 1740 to the 1850s, also saw considerable alteration to the landscape of Britain.

Workers no longer owned the tools of their trade. Industrial towns emerged with housing for workers which grew up around the factories and mills. Traditional apprenticeship systems existed where each master housed, fed and clothed as well as trained apprentices. Children, especially from the workhouses and orphanages, became part of the workforce.

The conditions of and hours of work for the working population, was marked by overwork, malnutrition and subsequent illness. Disease and death were the added ingredients to an environment where the pursuit of profits over rode concerns for health.

Occupational health during the nineteenth century was largely linked with parliamentary reforms and the Public Health Movement. The reforms spearheaded by the likes of Chadwick, Peel, Shaftesbury and Southwood-Smith contributed to creating the platform for further developments in the twentieth century.

1803 – The Health and Morals of Apprentices Act. This Act specifically related to parish apprentices in the cotton industry. Hours of work were limited to 12 hours per day; no work was to be undertaken between 9 am and 6 pm. Provisions for ventilation, whitewashing of premises, clothing, religious instruction and teaching reading, writing and arithmetic was encouraged. The Act in effect rested on the segregation of the sexes in the workplace.

1819 – First Factories Act. This Act forbade the employment of children under the age of nine. The hours of work were limited to 13.5 hours per day for those under 16 years. The enforcement of this legislation met with some difficulties as there was inadequate regulation of factories and a lack of inspectors.

1833 – Factories Act. There was specific reference in this legislation to the textile industry i.e. cotton, woollen, worsted, flax, hemp, tow and silk mills. The minimum age for the commencement of full employment was fixed for children at the age of nine. Working hours were limited to 48 hours per week for children aged between 9 and 14. After aged 14 and up to 18, the limit became 69 hours per week. Night work was strictly not permitted for those below the age of 18. Education was encouraged for children under 11 years. In addition to this development, Factory Inspectors were appointed to enforce this legislation. Doctors were also appointed to certify that children were fit for work and were aged nine upwards. These certifying medics became the forerunners of the later appointed factory doctors.

1842 – Mines Act. The act forbade the employment of girls, women and boys under the age of ten underground. There was no provision for school attendance. Mines inspectors were appointed.

1844 – Factories Act. Limited the hours of work for women and young persons to the age of 12. However, it reduced the minimum age of employment to eight. Hours of work for children were limited to 6.5 hours per day for those under the age of 13. Schooling was made compulsory for at least 3 hours per day.

1847 – Ten Hour Act. A 10 hour day was introduced for women and children under the age of 18.

1855 – Factory Act. This act gave medical officers new duties, function and powers to certify that young persons were not incapacitated for work by disease or bodily infirmity, and to investigate industrial accidents. These powers hailed the advent of a rudimentary industrial medical service, the first of its kind introduced by law in Great Britain. Regulations and periodic inspections were made in workplaces regarding lead paint, lucifer matches, explosives containing dinitro-benzene and those vulcanizing rubber with carbon disulphide and enamelling iron plates manufacture.

1860 – Mines Act. Raised the age for underground employment of boys to 12, however, exemption was allowed for those over the age of ten who produced certificates of literacy.

1864 – Factories (Extension Act). This act brought other industries within the scope of legislation. These included, paper staining, fustian cutting, pottery, match and cartridge manufacture.

1867 – Further Extension Act. Covered all industries with more than 50 employees.

1871 – Factories Act. Transferred responsibility for workshops to the Factory Inspectorate (this was formerly under the auspices of the local authority).

1880 – Employers' Liability Act. Enabled injured workmen to sue the employer who had to prove negligence (who had to prove that the employer had been negligent).

1895 – Notification of Diseases. A notification system was introduced which provided knowledge relating to industrial diseases. This was initially the case for lead and arsenic poisoning, as well as anthrax. Surgeons were empowered to suspend workers who were suffering as a result of accident or illness. The high prevalence of lead poisoning in the potteries and in white lead works, and the incidence of phossy jaw among the matchmakers, received a great deal of publicity.

The events, and the need to deal with notifications and reports from certifying surgeons, led to the subsequent appointment in 1898 of Thomas Legge (1863–1932). He became Medical Inspector of Factories and made over 30 years contribution to the service of occupational medicine, listing and preventing occupational disease. His main publication is *Industrial Maladies* published 2 years after his death in 1934.

1897 – Workman's Compensation Act. The employer was now liable for any accidents caused in the workplace regardless of the party or parties involved in negligence.

1906 – Workman's Compensation Act. This was extended to cover industrial diseases.

1925 – Workman's Compensation Act. Extended the list of industrial diseases.

1948 – National Insurance (Industrial Injuries) Act. The state took over responsibility for payment of benefit for all industrial injury and disease, regardless of consideration of negligence. The right was restored to the worker to sue at Common Law, in addition, recovering damages if he could prove employer's negligence. (Under the Workman's Compensation Act he had to chose between receiving payments under the Act and proceeding at Common Law).

Factories Acts were passed in 1937 (mainly a consolidating act) and short amending Acts in 1948, 1959 and 1961.

1954 – Mines and Quarries Act
1963 – Office, Shops and Railway Premises Act
1972 – Employment Medical Advisory Service Act
1974 – Health and Safety at Work etc., Act
1980 – Control of Lead at Work Regulations
1981 – Health and Safety (First Aid) Regulations
1983 – New Control Limits for Asbestos
1988 – Control of Substances Hazardous to Health Regulations
1994 – COSHH Amendments

1992 – New European legislation relating to: *Manual Handling – (Operating Regulations)*, *Visual Display Units*, *Managing Health and Safety*, *Display Screen Equipment*, *The Provision and Use of Work Equipment Regulations*, *The Workplace (Health Safety and Welfare Regulations)*, *Personal Protective Equipment at Work Regulations.*

These latter regulations are discussed in more detail in Chapter 3.

The work and health movement

Issues relating to occupational health and safety came from many perspectives. The following section is intended to outline some of the main influences of the movement from both popular and neglected perspectives.

The Chadwickian tradition

Edwin Chadwick took control of the sanitary movement in the 1830s and 1840s. His views emanated from a career in law and civil service, and he was a staunch supporter of Benthamite philosophy. For Chadwick, engineering was to be regarded as the hand maiden to the political economy of felicific calculus, in order to achieve the greatest happiness for the greatest number. Chadwick's movement stemmed from his personal beliefs which advocated that the science of engineering as opposed to medicine, was crucial to sanitary reform (a perspective also advocated by Virchow). However, it did not develop in the way he would have liked because from the beginning, public health was medically dominated.

Under the secretariat of the Poor Law Commission in 1838, Chadwick's colleagues employed three medical practitioners as inspectors to inquire into the state of health and sickness in London. Arnott, Kay-Shuttleworth and Southwood-Smith compiled a report which revealed the desperate living conditions of the poor in London.

The result of the Poor Law Commission Report of 1842 (published by Chadwick) underlined that epidemic diseases were caused by a dirty environment. The means of prevention was largely the provision of clean water supplies, effective sewerage and drainage, removal of nuisances such as refuse from the streets, roads, control of industrial effluent and the establishment of new standards of environmental and personal cleanliness.

The report specifically outlined a new structure of administration which included the appointment of medical officers for each district to inspect and report on local sanitary conditions. Soon after, the Royal Commission in 1843 was set up to consider the health of towns. The consequence was the passing of the Public Health Act of 1848 which established the General Board of Health, and the co-ordination of municipal responsibilities for environmental regulation.

The importance of education and propaganda in achieving the purposes of public health had its origins in the UK. It was in the Chadwickian tradition that the emergence of messages relating to health improvement came about. Indeed, it was highlighted by the Metropolitan Health of Towns Association formed in 1844:

... to diffuse among the people the valuable information elicited by recent enquiries, and the advancement of science, as to the physical and moral evils that result from the present defective sewerage, drainage of water supply, air and light and construction of dwelling houses

Sutherland 1987, p. 5

In addition to these values, Southwood- Smith wrote a pamphlet prior to his appointment as medical officer on the General Board of Health. Its title was: *An Address to the Working Classes of the United Kingdom on Their Duty to the Present State of the Sanitary Question*. It was from this time onwards, a minor step to alter a tract or a pamphlet into a poster, leaflet or an exhibition, or even lecture, was made to communicate a message. These became the tool of doctors such as Kingsley who developed a great enthusiasm for health education.

Despite such enthusiasm, however, health propagandism was slow to take hold. Initially, it formed a great link with the Victorian notion of individual charity. Later, industrialists such as Rowntree, Cadbury and Owen took on the importance of health of the workforce in their public and private domains. For example, to encourage the development of a better work environment, it was activity undertaken aside from daily toil which improved worker relations, especially the youth:

Encouraging an amenable work environment
... the employees have the use of a considerable portion of the grounds surrounding the Works, and in fine weather the lawns and gardens attract many of them, especially the younger girls, who play cricket and other games. Or for those who stay indoors, newspapers, games, such as dominoes, draughts, etc., are provided in the dining-rooms, and occasionally concerts and meetings are held.

Rowntree & Co., 1916, p. 16

Women made their mark in the development of health education during the public health movement. Manchester claims to have invented health visiting because the ladies section of the Manchester and Salford Sanitary Association employed women of the working class to visit poorer people and teach them the laws of health as early as 1862.

In 1890, the Manchester Corporation agreed to pay the salaries of six of the city's 14 health visitors. By 1905, a trained female supervisor was appointed and later nurses began to do the job. The developments gained some momentum in selected parts of the country and also saw the appointment of the first health visitor in Liverpool in 1897, and Birmingham in 1899. Some of the work relating to the reduction of infant mortality was extended further in such progressive areas as Huddersfield. By 1905, Longwood District, Huddersfield, all children reaching their first birthday during that year received a gift of £1. Doctors were encouraged to notify births, setting up pure milk distribution depots and the establishment of experimental day nurseries for working mothers. Additional health information was also provided for new mothers concerning the 'golden rules' for child and mother care.

Progress in these developments, alongside reports relating to the effects of poverty on health prompted legislation which for the first time linked health and education. Under the auspices of Rowntree, Newman and Booth, the 1907 Education (Administrative Provisions) Act saw the erection of a national system of supervision of the health of children.

Concern for the health of young women
The ... Procedure is followed in the case of girls. It is felt that the change from school life to factory life for girls of 14 and 15 years of age is a time of both physical and intellectual strain, and that it is necessary that special care should be given to a young girl to ensure her development into a healthy, intelligent, and skilful worker. All girls are therefore engaged by a member of the social staff, and all who are under 16 are put in the 'follow-up' reports ... the consequence is that a young girl entering the Factory feels that someone is interested in how she gets on with her work; her health is watched, and advice given on this and other matters, and she is thus helped through the critical months of industrial life

Rowntree & Co., 1916, p. 12

Although legislation was passed, health propaganda remained largely on the periphery of professional interest. Industry and the unions remained largely uncommitted from the end of Victoria's reign to the end of the second world war. Central government, despite all the legislation which might have been relevant but was not (i.e. Ministry of Health Act 1918, Local Government Act 1929, the Education Act 1944, and the National Health Service Act 1946) remained in administrative conflict with local authorities. In essence, both were not interested (Sutherland 1987).

Engels' observations

Engels discusses, often in graphic detail, the problems of work and its impact on health amongst the working classes and abhors the effect of capitalism in the nineteenth century. He not only underlines the problems for people in the workplace, he characteristically discusses some of the problems that can and did extend into the home and the social environment, providing a richness and a potence to the hard, dull and cruel lives of the poor and working classes. In his most noted work on the subject, *The Conditions of the Working Class in England*, Engels' theoretical position was unambiguous. For working class people, the root of illness and early death lay in the organisation of economic production and in the social environment.

In his observations of what he considered to be the realities of British capitalism, working people were forced to live and work within circumstances that led to ill health. He demonstrated through a series of descriptions, how this became the case. Engels' analysis of alcoholism came in an account of the social milieu that fostered excessive consumption of alcohol. Alcoholism became a response to the problems of working class life. Workers turned to alcohol as a substitute for the absence of emotional gratification. Engels regarded this situation as the responsibility of the capitalists. Indeed, he makes known that

> Liquor is their only source of pleasure ... the working man ... must have something to make work worth his trouble, to make the prospect of the next day endurable ... drunkenness has here ceased to be a vice for which the vicious can be held responsible ... they who have degraded the working man to a mere object have the responsibility to bear.
>
> Engels 1845, pp. 141–142

It is interesting that these observations of the nineteenth century are still pertinent at the close of the twentieth century in terms of the plight of the ordinary working person, as highlighted in *The Guardian, 3rd June 1998:*

... why must we still yearn to be the global top-dog? Can't we just accept ourselves for what we are – a medium sized country that has long since said goodbye to its empire and much of its manufacturing industry? For all this talk of modernisation, as I've pointed out before, Blair actually wants to propel us back to the nineteenth century as quickly as possible, with a stern programme of self-help, thrift, clean living and muscular Christianity, Gradgrinian education and plenty of hard labour. Would he have quite so much Stakhanovite zeal if he were a 24 year old stacking supermarket shelves or cleaning office floors for a princely £3.20 an hour?

The main difference from the nineteenth century is that it is not only the working classes that are proletarianised:

... well paid executives ... feel thoroughly enslaved by their work. A survey carried out by the EFD consultancy, and published ... in Management Today, found that about half (52.5 per cent) of its 5,500 respondents spent between 41 and 50 hours at work every week, and a further quarter (26.2 per cent) averaged more than 51 hours. Most regretted that they seldom saw their children or spouses; some had even missed the birth of their own babies because of pressure of work; one man had had to postpone his father's funeral. Nearly half said that professional commitments were wrecking their private and social lives. In short, the nation already has its shoulder to the wheel – and is cracking under the strain ....

Society, Wheen 1998, G2, p. 5

The Engellian society saw alcohol as rooted firmly within the social structure. The view posited by Engels emphasised that deprivation and poor social conditions should be changed to enable all to participate equally and fairly in society. Basic treatment programmes focussing on the individual were, in his view, not going to solve poverty and inequity in society.

Industrial accidents were an additional source of concern. For Engels, accidents were particularly marked in the case of machinery. The most common accidents involved loss of fingers, hands or arms by contact with unguarded machines. Engels also pointed to orthopaedic disorders derived from the physical demands of industrialism. He identified that the curvature of the spine, deformities of the lower extremities, flat feet, varicose veins and leg ulcers as manifestations of work demands that required long periods of time in an upright posture. Engels also discussed the health effects on posture, standing and repetitive movements:

All these afflictions are easily explained by the nature of factory work ... the operatives ... must stand the whole time. And one who sits down, say upon a window ledge or a basket, is fined, and this perpetual upright position, the constant mechanical pressure of the upper positions of the body upon spinal column, hips and legs, inevitably produces the results mentioned. This standing is not required by the work itself ....

pp. 190–193

Advocates of Engels' position, such as Waitzkin, also emphasize that although musculoskeletal disorders, accidents and deprivation, exposure to toxic substances were a main source of illness at work. It was not, however, until the 1970s, that serious attention was paid to such issues.

Lace making is still done by hand today in large measure, and predominantly by women. Albeit, machinery for this process has been available since 1808. Engels observations led him to describe some of the realities of the industry and the impact on health of workers in Nottingham and Leicester, UK:

The work is very bad for the eyes, and although a permanent injury in the case of threaders is not universally observable, inflammation of the eye, pain, tears and momentary uncertainty of vision during the act of threading are engendered. For the winders, however, it is certain that their work seriously affects the eye and produces, besides the frequent inflammations of the cornea, many cases of decay of vision and cataract.

p. 205

Children were also subject to conditions that endangered their health. Indeed, Engels goes on to cite the Children's Employment Commission's report of the period where children working in lace factories are subject to the most difficult conditions. Most of all is the

... unwholesome ... work of the runners, who are usually children of 7, and even of 5 and 4 years old. Commissioner Grainger actually found one child of 2 years old employed at this work. Following a thread which is to be withdrawn by a needle from an intricate texture, is very bad for the eyes, especially when, as is usually the case, the work is continued 14 to 16 hours. In the least unfavourable case, aggravated near sightedness follows; in the worst case, which is frequent enough, incurable blindness from decay of vision.

p. 206

Lead poisoning was also another issue that Engels had come upon in his travels. However, issues relating to the health impact of the pottery industry was not given any great attention until the latter part of the nineteenth century, some 40 years after Engels' communications. This issue was underlined by Waitzkin (1981) in that:

The consequences Engels described include severe abdominal pain, constipation and neurologic complications like epilepsy and partial or complete paralysis. These signs of lead intoxication occurred not only in workers themselves, according to Engels, but also in children who lived near pottery factories. Epidemiologic evidence concerning the community hazards of industrial lead has gained attention in environmental health mainly since 1970, again without recognition of Engels' observations.

p. 82

Engels also discusses diseases contracted in:

1   the textile industry of 'brown lung' or byssinosis;
2   manufacturing of knives and forks, i.e. 'Grinders asthma', a respiratory disease contracted by inhaling metallic dust; and
3   coal mining, i.e. 'Black spittle' now called 'black lung' or pneumoconiosis.

Engels emphasised that the majority, if not all of these conditions could be prevented by illustrating the contradiction between profit and adequate health conditions in capitalist industry:

Every case of this disease ends fatally ... in all the coal mines which are properly ventilated this disease is unknown, while it frequently happens that miners who go from well to ill ventilated mines are seized by it. The profit greed of mine owners which prevents the use of ventilators is therefore responsible for the fact that this working men's disease exists at all.

p. 279

There is frequently talk of the feminist perspective as a missing element in workplace health of the past. This is not true. Barbara Harrison's (1996) sterling work on working women between 1880 and 1914 makes the issues more apparent, however, Engels told us sometimes in rather graphic detail, even exhibiting a ferocious anger at their plight. The issues of deprivation and exploitation are clearly marked out in his work. Gender roles, family life, mortality and morbidity, conditions for women and children are all apparent.

Women at work were often exploited at high cost to their health.

> Women often return to the mill 3 or 4 days after confinement, leaving the baby of course; in the dinner hour they must hurry home to feed the child and eat something, and what sort of suckling that can be is also evident. Lord Ashley repeats the testimony of several workmen: M.H., 20 years old, has two children, the youngest a baby, that is tended by the other, a little older. The mother goes to the mill shortly after five o'clock in the morning, and comes home at eight at night; all day the milk pours from her breasts, so that her clothing drips with it. H.W. has three children, goes away Monday morning at five o'clock and comes back Saturday evening; has so much to do for the children then that she cannot go to bed before three o'clock in the morning; often wet through to the skin, and obliged to work in that state. She said: 'My breasts have given me the most frightful pain, and I have been dripping with milk'.
>
> Engels 1845, p. 166

Another observation of women's bodies is marked in the corporeal reality through the impact of work and working conditions.

> 1   The influence of factory work upon the female physique also is marked and peculiar. The deformities entailed by long hours of work are much more serious among men. Protracted work frequently causes deformities of the pelvis, partly in the shape of abnormal position and development of the hip bones, partly of malformation of the lower portion of the spinal column. (Engels, p. 179); and
> 2   That factory operatives undergo more difficult confinement than other women is testified to by several midwives and accoucheurs, and also that they are more liable to miscarriage. Moreover, they suffer from the general enfeeblement common to all operatives, and when pregnant, continue to work in the factory up to the hour of delivery because otherwise they lose their wages and are made to fear that they may be replaced if they stop away too soon. It frequently happens that women are at work evening and delivered the next morning, and the case is none too rare of their being delivered in the factory among the machinery ....
>
> Engels 1845, pp. 179–180

In many cases the family was not wholly dissolved by the employment of the wife, but rather demonstrated a reversal of role out of necessity. The wife supported the family, the husband, if he remained with his family rather than straying, was at home tending to children, sweeping the rooms and acting as cook. Engels recounted (around 1843) a situation of a working man visiting an old friend in St. Helen's Lancashire.

> ... He found him in a miserable, damp cellar, scarcely furnished; and when my poor friend went in, there sat poor Jack near the fire and what did he think of you? Why he sat and mended his wife's stockings with the bodkin; and as soon as he saw his old friend at the doorpost, he tried to hide them. But Joe, that is my friend's name, had seen it and said: 'Jack, what the devil art thou doing? Where is the missions? Why? Is that thy work?' And poor Jack was ashamed, and said: 'No, I know this is not my work, but my poor missus is i' th' factory; she has to leave at half past five and works till eight at night, and then she is so knocked up that she cannot do ought when she gets home, so I have to do everything for her what I can, for I have no work, nor had any for more nor 3 years and I shall never have any more work while I live'; and he wept a big tear. Jack again said: 'there is work enough for women folks and children hereabouts, but none for men; thou mayest sooner find a hundred pound on the road than work for men – but I should never have believed that either thou or anyone else would have seen me mending my wife's stockings, for it is bad work. But she can hardly stand on her feet ...'
>
> Engels 1845, pp. 167–168

Engels analysis of the social origins of illness was part of a much broader agenda. Like other Marxist scholarship, his book was intended mainly for the purpose of the sociopolitical action. Engels quickly focussed on additional theoretical and practical concerns. Despite later writings on natural and physical sciences, he did not return to the social origins of illness as a major issue in its own right. Yet in a book that aimed toward a broad description of working class life, Engels provided clear analysis of the causal relationship between social structure and physical illness.

After Engels, the 1890s saw a rise in a substantial literature on the effects of industrial efficiency. It was acknowledged that industrial work lead to deafness, skin conditions, fractures, back pain, hernias due to lifting heavy loads, arthritis, rheumatism and varieties of poisoning as a result of toxic substances (Weindling 1985).

The use of statistics and stories describing accidents and diseases experienced by workers was rarely used as an indicator of the wider social conditions. According to Weindling (1985), a good deal could be learned from medical institutions, dispensaries and welfare clinics for outpatients who suffered such conditions. There was also limited long term studies of sickness related to industrial work. The early work undertaken by doctors, even in routine cases, is also a missing element in piecing together the evidence from this period.

The Rosen, Sigerist and Teleky influences

By the end of the nineteenth century, legislation was actively mobilised to protect mainly children and women from factors leading to ill health in the work place. Also, the Public Health Movement in Britain had identified a multifaceted approach to improving health not only through the politico-legal system, but also through the medical and nursing professions as well as propaganda. This was followed early into the twentieth century under the guidance and leadership of Newman. However, another strand of the work-place health movement was unfolding in Germany and America.

Despite a series of political and war time setbacks, the field of workplace health began to develop. It was upgraded as an academic specialism in post graduate education during the 1920s and for the most part, has taken a scientific emphasis, although this has altered in the latter part of the twentieth century to include health promotion. The social strand owes much to the efforts of Rosen, Sigerist and Teleky.

Henry Sigerist with his followers, attempted to reorient medicine to social problems by emphasizing the social history of medicine from the patient's perspective. (It is interesting that we have to wait until the end of the twentieth century for the lay perspective to become valid in the field of health / professions allied to medicine research). Sigerist campaigned in Leipzig and John Hopkins Universities. He also campaigned for industrial health insurance schemes. By 1937 he predicted that the 'New History' of social conditions and culture, combined with the awareness of the importance of social medicine, would result in a development of the history of occupational medicine.

George Rosen was of similar attitude when he visited Germany. He became impressed by attitudes towards occupational health and so called for the history of occupational medicine to become a major branch of history.

The impetus came during the 1920s to restore social and political dimensions to occupational medicine by the first medical inspector, Thomas Legge and the pioneer of social medicine *Ludvig Teleky*.

Influenced by Marx in his early writings, his theoretical discussion of occupational health demanded that the historian and scholar recognized the centrality of economic structure and incorporated the activities of the working class in medical history. The history of occupational health was pivotal to Rosen because occupational diseases were so evidently caused by social circumstances (Rosen 1937). He stressed that diseases are not immutable entities and are intelligible only within their biological and social contexts, and he suggested that history of medicine had been deficient in viewing the patient as 'only an accident of the history of disease'.

Rosen made this argument in order to demonstrate to doctors that their endeavour was necessarily social. He wanted to show that the most astute physicians were those who understood the social aetiology of disease and that the most successful healers were those who acted on this premise. There was, however, one further lesson that Rosen proposed for doctors who granted this point. This was to recognize the necessity of becoming a social critic. Through his early work on occupational medicine and the role of the physician, Rosen was germinating the concept of social medicine that he articulated in the years immediately following World War Two.

Just as Rosen denied that Marx was a strict economic determinist, he also looked at other cultural elements in explaining the development of healthcare. In his efforts to demonstrate that medicine could not be understood outside of the broad social context, Rosen was willing to invoke the power of ideas as much as the means of production.

Rosen's campaign was to reorient attitudes, along with the campaigns by Sigerist for socialised medicine, by condemning the focussed attention of scientific advances in physiology and toxicology. His ideal position was to advocate the study of occupational diseases within a social context, thus bringing forth new ideological perspectives. This in turn, may have contributed to solving some of the difficulties identified in occupational medicine, and so developing an understanding of the broader social contexts in which disease is contracted and developed. However, his ideals were not yet to be achieved, as despite his publications in the field, the world remained silent on social occupational medicine. Social medicine, generally lost its significance during the Second World War. It was not until the latter part of the 1960s, and early 1970s that others such as Gardell take up the mantle (see Chapter 6).

Ludwig Teleky's main focus for concern rested on the reform of social insurance. For the most part, he devised an effective method to reduce health risks and improve worker safety with the aid of insurance. His observations relied on the premise that social security organisations would express their discontent if employers were made liable for general damage to health. He considered the benefits of introducing a sliding tariff for contributions of the employers to social insurance, according to the frequency of accidents occurring in their factories. Teleky believed that this, rather than the general hygiene or technical requirements would result in more direct improvements in worker safety. He was also of the notion that workers would gain greater benefit if illness was proven as a result of occupation. This would stimulate greater criteria for compensation and initiatives involving prevention. Benefit could also be gained through insurance against accidents as opposed to compensation as a result of disability.

Teleky proposed automatic liability from accident insurance as soon as an accident took place. Such a regulation, he maintained, could be achieved by the drawing up of a comprehensive register of occupational diseases. Teleky's propositions sought to improve the position of the employee and at the same time, triggered forces into the prevention of ill health in the workplace, hence elevating the field of industrial hygiene.

Teleky's ideals became realised in the Occupational Disease Act in 1925. However, only marginal improvements were made for those few who were affected.

The contribution of the trades unions

It was not until 1924 that there came a significant Trades Union Congress (TUC) publication which presented its initial concern for worker health. *The Waste of Capitalism* stated clearly that workers should take control of the work environment and also challenged the value of joint negotiating committees where workers had no real power.

However, the unions were not yet to have their glory as the General Strike of the 1920s and 1930s, together with mass unemployment, fragmented union activity and organisation. Indeed, membership fell considerably from 37.6 per cent to 23.9 per cent of the total workforce. Participation in national activity also fell, whilst leadership became more bureaucratic.

Trade union leaders became wary of preventive health and safety schemes for fear that they would increase unemployment, emphasizing instead, hazard pay and increased compensation benefits for employees. Compensation was seen as a visible attack on many dangerous working practices and conditions.

Between the years of the TUC publication and the early part of the 1950s, there was little work undertaken in formulating a strategy for prevention. In fact in 1934, Thomas Legge, who retired from the Factory Inspectorate over the government's refusal to ratify the Geneva White Lead Convention, said of asbestosis: 'Looking back in the light of present knowledge, it is impossible not to feel that opportunities for discovery and prevention were badly missed'. (Clutterbuck 1980).

Many cases of cadmium poisoning had been reported, but it was not to be a recognized occupational disease until 1953. Beta-naphthylanine was also known as long ago as 1895 to cause bladder cancer, but the Imperial Chemical Industries (ICI) continued to produce it. They were eventually fined £20,000 but even 85 years later, it is recognized that all people who were exposed have not been contacted and checked.

Polyvinyl chloride (PVC) plastic is also an example of a substance which was manufactured without any attention to its potential damage to health. It was not until 1995 that voluntary environmental controls were established by the European Council for Vinyl Manufacturers. It has been known to be carcinogenic since the 1970s (Viola et al. 1971). So Legge had a point. These issues were treated rather too cautiously as far as employee protection was concerned.

Interest came from the Labour Party and the TUC in relation to the development of a co-ordinated occupational health service in the 1940s. However, this was consistently blocked by the government. This is despite the setting up of an Industrial Health Research Board directed by the Medical Research Council (MRC). It established units on pneumoconiosis (1945), toxicology (1947) and pollution (1955), and at a number of universities. The end of the war saw a rise in union membership again and heralded a more persistent approach to the subject of worker health and safety at a series of TUC conferences.

By 1954, a motion was forwarded urging the government to mobilize strategies towards accident prevention. This would have included setting up committees in industrial and non-industrial forums. The resolution was withdrawn when the General Council argued that it might reduce the employers' liability for accidents, thus creating a smokescreen without any intention of carrying out the necessary work.

Prior to becoming Chair of the Health and Safety Commission, Bill Simpson, of the Foundry Workers section of the Amalgamated Union of Engineering Workers, was responsible for organising, campaigning for and training in issues of safety. Rights for safety representatives were won under the Mines and Quarries Act in 1954. However, it was not until 1961 that further regulations under the Factory Act were issued. These included pulling together existing legislation and established minimum standards for institutions recognised as traditional factories. This rested largely on lighting, heating, ventilation, cleaning, guarding and fire procedures.

Despite this amalgamation, there is little evidence to indicate that health and safety legislation was a result of union pressure. For the most part, it came from the shop floor. Indeed, a mass of evidence was presented on workers behalf through companies, industrial associations, the TUC and CBI to the Robens Committee in 1970.

Robens' recommendations and philosophy served as the basis of the new Health and Safety at Work etc., Act of 1974. Unfortunately, Robens saw no need for an occupational health service, and blamed employers for their own misfortune in the workplace through apathy.

Nichols' (1990) analysis of accident statistics of the late 1970s to the early 1980s indicated that trade union training was a positive contribution to health and safety movement at work. Indeed, Walters and Gourlay (1990) found that union contribution came firstly, through the provision of a positive relationship between central trade union organization and effective representation. Secondly, the integration of effective safety representatives into the workplace organisation of the trade unions. Thirdly, the importance of information and particularly training for effective safety representatives. Fourthly, the importance of consultation between the safety representatives and the constituencies they represent. Finally, the overwhelming importance of management's commitment to taking seriously both health and safety and employee participation (Walters 1990).

Occupational health development, UK

In the UK, concern over the health of women munitions workers (Theson and Thom 1983) provided the background to establishing the Industrial Fatigue Research Board. The Medical Research Council assumed responsibility for this Committee, which became the Industrial Health Research Board in 1928. Although largely a period of development and scientific experimentation, particularly for Charles Sherrington and the Haldanes, it was silicosis research conducted by Donald Hunter that yielded the rewards of a research department in 1943, at the London School of Hygiene.

The wartime improvements that were undertaken in occupational health and social medicine, however, failed to culminate in a state occupational health service. There were a few studies of note in occupational medicine which alerted to ways of addressing some problems. For example, the Glasgow expert in public health, Thomas Ferguson, made substantial contributions to the impact of industrial work on sickness in Scotland. Andrew Meiklejohn, a specialist in silicosis, had a keen sense of how history was relevant to the problems experienced in occupational medicine. He demonstrated how since the 1930s the shift in research on silicosis, from physiological approaches to the recognition that it was caused by dust rather than muscular exertion, marked a return to views of the 1860s. His recognition of the contributions of Thomas Percival of an earlier period were still reflected in his views in the 1950s.

Founding departments of occupational medicine

The development of occupational medicine in the UK has been largely on a voluntary basis, either by large companies, or later nationalized industries. The first department, although short lived, was founded in Birmingham.

The Association of Industrial Medical Officers inaugurated in 1935, had 21 founder members. The 1939–1945 war heralded emergency legislation covering factories. This continued after the war despite the fact that conflicts arose and ensued between the interests of industrial medical officers and general practitioners, who were performing statutory duties of a certifying surgeon.

It was on 25th June 1940, that Bevin's policy was accepted that the factory inspectorate should require that larger factories appoint a medical officer, nurses and first aid staff to supervise health and welfare. Smaller places of work were left without provision, although the late 1940s saw pioneering experiments at Slough, Central Middlesex, Harlow in the USA at New Haven for small firms to share medical facilities.

The Nuffield foundation set up by motor magnate Lord Nuffield, provided initial finances for setting up non-profit making companies to provide, on a capitation fee basis, medical and nursing care at work for employees of small and medium sized firms. Industries that benefited from this patronage included those situated in: Slough (1947), Harlow New Town (1955), Central Middlesex (1956), Rochdale (1962), Dundee (1962), West Midlands (1963), and the North of England (1960). In more recent years, new towns such as Newton Aycliff, Telford and Milton Keynes (1984) have also benefited. Some 120,000 employees were covered under this scheme.

The route to developing a comprehensive service

Barriers to the development of an occupational health service in the UK on a national basis were largely due to the division of health responsibilities between ministries. Despite the energy of the Ministry of Labour under Bevan in expanding services post World War II, integration with the health service was not readily achieved. Thus, from the beginning, occupational health services rested in the hands of entrepreneurs almost spanning two centuries, with little or no regulation except through necessity.

It was during the 1950s that the Trades Union Congress (TUC) brought pressure to further stimulate interest in occupational health in the Ministry of Labour. This was not without difficulty as there was a requirement for the government to balance welfare expenditure against proposed tax cuts. Also, there were problems concerning regulation of standards, largely due to the adhoc manner in which the service began and was sustained in some areas. This unevenness of provision was not to alter until the establishment of the Health and Safety Executive in 1974.

In 1954, the Dale Committee report concluded in its findings that the existing state of industrial health services could no longer continue. The provision of medical treatment and care was seen as largely inadequate for industry as a whole. The committee called for more comprehensive provision. Unfortunately, this was never taken up by the government.

By 1961, The British Medical Association (BMA) Working Party (Alexander Report) and the Porritt Committee 1962, urged the government to set up a comprehensive occupational health service under the NHS Area Health Boards. The Report stated that:

... the National Health Service should be responsible through area health boards for running all medical services including preventive and social health services and occupational health services covering industry and commerce.

Tyrer and Lee 1984, p. 17

It soon became apparent that there was no government response to the Committees requests. By May 1970, the Secretary of State for Employment and Productivity set up a Committee to enquire into the provisions made for the safety and health of persons in employment (this excluded transport workers).

The Committee headed by Lord Robens reported in 1972, was followed by the Health and Safety at Work etc., Act 1974. This was despite the fact that Robens was extremely critical of some of the existing industrial medical services. It was underlined that doctors were duplicating facilities which should be provided by the NHS, especially in the field of accident and emergency.

The Committee stated that specialist skills were required which differed in range from general medical care. Statutory provision was also limited. These duties were carried out by up to 1300 appointed factory doctors, the majority being general practitioners without occupational training. The main duties included:

1 the examination of young people entering employment from school;
2 the examination of workers in processes covered by regulations; and
3 the investigation of gassing accidents and industrial diseases to confirm diagnosis.

They were the successors to the original examining surgeons in the nineteenth century.

The Employment Medical Advisory Service (EMAS)

Although an Employment Medical Advisory Service (EMAS) was recommended by the Robens Committee, largely in terms of a foundation of occupational medicine for the country, it did not recommend that the government should involve itself further in the provision of an occupational health service.

EMAS, established in 1973, was the body responsible for the removal of medical inspectors from the factory inspectorate and used them to form the nucleus of the new advisory service under a separate administration within the Department of Employment. Today it is called the Medical Division of the Health and Safety Executive.

The Medical Division has the powers to investigate and advise on any health problem appearing to be related to employment at the request of:

- the employer/manager
- employee
- trade union
- factory inspector
- doctor in general practice/hospital/public health
- disablement resettlement officer
- teacher/parent/individual initiative
- careers officer

The Medical Division has also assumed responsibility for the medical supervision of workers attending government employment rehabilitation centres. This was considered ample replacement for general practitioners formerly employed on a sessional basis. Advice and support is also provided for resettlement officers with cases where the effect of disability on working capacity was in question (as there were no medical reports available concerning the disabled).

The body has also held responsibility for the initiation of and carrying out epidemiological research, either alone or in collaboration with appropriate research bodies. The service covers the nation and advises voluntary services in setting up occupational health services; its mainly a consultant service, investing time in investigating specific problems.

By 1983, the services were still inequitable and fragmented. The House of Lords Select Committee on Science and Technology conducted an enquiry under the chairmanship of Lord Gregson into the future of occupational health and hygiene services. The Gregson report was published in 1983. They found that the service for employees in the NHS was extensive, but rudimentary. Provision for small firms was minimal.

The Committee underlined the necessity of the extension of occupational health services for medium and smaller companies. Early detection of hazards at work was considered important as it would alleviate suffering for affected employees and reduce the financial burden on the employer and state. To achieve its aims, the Committee recognised that training of doctors and nurses would have to be an integral aspect of their strategy.

Such a step was, unfortunately not undertaken as it required statutory support from the government. The government was reluctant to commit itself firstly because it would create demand for trained personnel greater than the supply available. Secondly, it would impose unwelcome and sudden additional costs to industry and finally, would provoke hostility and resentment where co-operation and sympathy are crucial. There was the additional burden of increased bureaucracy, as well as there being insufficient flexibility for varying needs (see Chapter 6 for current issues).

The workplace health movement outlined so far, has seen the conflicts and tensions that have existed between interested parties. The overwhelming evidence suggests the issue of health is at the centre of these developments and yet still in terms of advancement along the road towards improvement which has been difficult as far as the needs of the workforce are concerned. Bodies have emerged in a fragmented way and hence their influences have largely centred upon the main issue, yet at the same time beset with problems beyond their control, namely, the political and economic climates, and whether such issues are suitable for attention in the public domain at the time. The following chapters extend knowledge of the developments in the workplace health movement.

Chapter 3

Regulatory developments, roles and functions

This chapter is intended to broadly outline the historico-political dimensions which impinged upon the formation of a service for workplace health improvement. It also assesses the roles and functions of services to maintain health as well as the legal requirements and their implications for managers and employees. The chapter ends with discussion on more recent initiatives on the workplace health movement at the approach of the millennium.

As discussed in the earlier chapters, problems related to health in the workplace have a long history. The need for and development of an occupational health service or at least a service that attended to the needs of employees' well being was a necessary development. Surprisingly then, despite the advancement of industry in all sectors, including technology, the needs of those at the forefront of change and productivity, the workers, was not paramount. History has taught us that it is through necessity and struggle that the worker can ever achieve, whether collectively or as individuals.

A framework for health improvement

It was not until 1959 that we see the beginnings of a framework to introduce a service that provided for the health needs of workers. The field of occupational medicine had began to grow and expand driving the impetus towards the notion of an occupational health service.

Indeed, the aims of occupational health services as identified by the ILO in recommendation No. 112, was stated to be:

1   Contributing to workers' physical and mental adjustment in particular by adaptation of the work to the workers and their assignment to jobs for which they are suited. Hence some consideration to the ergonomic notion of fitting the job to the worker and a process of selection dependent on suitability, meaning skill.

2   Protection of workers against health hazards arising from the work or working conditions. The emphasis on safety was paramount in this statement.

3   Contributing to the establishment and maintenance of the highest possi-

ble degree of physical and mental well being. These broad general terms, are however, interpreted rather widely depending on the economic and social circumstances in each member country.

In Britain, a series of investigations into services to improve workers' health had been undertaken. Prior to the ILO recommendations outlined above, the Dale Committee (1954) found that industrial health services, although many were voluntary in terms of provision of care and treatment, could not continue in their present state. In fact, the service provision was rather poor and inadequate for the entire industry. The Committee called for a comprehensive provision of service across the country. Their recommendations were never taken up by the government of the time.

This was despite the fact that the enquiry had produced an outline of the working hours that medical officers had allocated to their duties in industry. In 1944, there were 180 full time doctors engaged in industry. This figure had plummeted to 51 in 1951. Of those operating on a part time basis, 339 were working between 3 and 12 hours per week in industry and 1,397 were working for 3 hours or less (Committee Enquiry 1951).

Missed opportunities

The reasons for such apathy in the role of industrial medicine is unclear. The issue of education and training had already been tackled by the BMA during the 1940s. By 1944, activity in this area was thriving as Merewether (1945, pp. 45–46) describes

The increase in appreciation of the importance of Industrial Health is evident in many ways and is widespread. The Royal College of Physicians has issued a valuable report on the subject, the TUC a statement and a resolution, the Universities of Durham, Glasgow and Manchester are in process of establishing Departments of Industrial Health with the assistance of substantial grants from the Nuffield foundation ... The Society of Apothecaries is taking steps to institute a Diploma in Industrial Health. The MRC has set up a Research Unit at Cardiff to study pneumoconiosis in coal miners ... the MRC's Department of Industrial Health Research at the London Hospital is actively prosecuting research. The Universities of Bristol, Leeds, Sheffield and Manchester with the London School of Hygiene and The Birmingham Accident Hospital provide brief courses ... in Industrial Health ... It is my belief that ... the healthiness or otherwise of an occupation will become increasingly the dominant factor in the choice of an occupation. Inescapably, therefore, unhealthy occupations must be made healthy or they will languish and ultimately fade out from lack of labour.

The evidence presented does not give much indication concerning the reasons for neglecting the incorporation of industrial health matters into the *NHS White Paper* of 1944. At best, it transpires that Bevin perceived industrial medicine to be concerned with the preventative, as opposed to being a personal medical service (Waldron 1996). Later evidence insists that this premise was largely a smokescreen, as in office Bevin took over responsibility for the Factories Department and was equally determined to keep industrial medicine away from the Ministry of Health: he linked them to the Factory Inspectorate (Watkins 1982).

By 1961, the BMA Working Party (Alexander Report) and the Porritt Committee 1962, urged the government to set up a comprehensive occupational health service under the NHS Area Health Boards. The report stated:

> The National Health Service should be responsible through area health boards for running all medical services including preventative and social health services and occupational health services covering industry and commerce.
>
> Tyrer and Lee 1982, p. 17

The Appointed Factory Doctor Service (AFDS) was examined by another body, which was a sub-committee of the Industrial Health Advisory Committee which recommended the AFDS replacement for a more expert service (HMSO 1966). This did not arrive until 1972 in the form of the Employment Medical Advisory Service (EMAS).

By May 1970, the Secretary of State for Employment and Productivity set up a Committee to enquire into the provisions made for the safety and health of persons in employment (with the exception of transport workers). The Committee, headed by Lord Robens, reported in 1972. It was followed by the Health and Safety at Work etc., Act 1974. The Robens Committee was critical of some of the existing industrial medical services, i.e. doctors thought to be duplicating facilities which should be provided by the NHS.

The Committee also reported that too much time was spent on casualty work and treatment. It identified that specialist skills were required which was not synonymous with general medical care. Praise was levied concerning recommendations for an employment medical advisory service, however, it was seen as a foundation of occupational medicine for the country and did not recommend that the government should involve itself further in the provision of an occupational health service.

EMAS was the brainchild of Trevor Lloyd Davies, who was the last Chief Medical Inspector, and whose ambition it was to provide for the first time in Britain a national focus for the development of occupational medicine. Although the necessity for a national occupational health service was underlined by the CBI, very little attention was given to the development of such a service. Priority was given to developing a comprehensive medical service instead.

EMAS assumed responsibility for the medical supervision of workers attending government employment rehabilitation centres and government training centres (now known as skills centres). This replaced general practitioners who were formerly employed on a sessional basis. Services of a medical nature for resettlement officers were provided with cases where effect of disability on working capacity was in question. The sector also held responsibility for the initiation of and carrying out epidemiological research, either alone or in collaboration with appropriate research bodies. The service covers the nation and advises voluntary services in setting up occupational health services.

The occupational health service

Over a period of almost 30 years, the system of occupational health has been shaped and re-shaped by policy influences and research with the field. It has moved from a safety and disease focus, to an emphasis on prevention with the advent of stress and the need to manage it at the end of the 1990s.

The original intentions for occupational health were outlined by the WHO in 1975, however, it has taken a considerable time to realise its ambitions. The universal definition of occupational health became known as:

1 the identification and subsequent control at the workplace of all known or suspected substances, agents and mechanisms that can lead to harm. This may be physical, chemical, biological and psychological agents;
2 to ensure that employees are fit to pursue employment. That is to say, having the physiological, anatomical, psychological and individual capacities to pursue work, and at the same time be aware of their limitations;
3 to provide mechanisms to protect those who may be vulnerable to adverse working conditions.

This has largely involved education of managers and their allies and health monitoring. (Health of the Nation Taskforce 1993).

It is interesting to note that two years earlier, its main responsibilities as identified by the same body included:

• identifying and controlling known or suspected work factors that contribute to ill health.
• educating management and workers to fulfil their responsibilities for health.
• promoting health programmes not primarily concerned with work related injury or disease.

The fact that the service has largely focussed, in Britain, on the first two aspects of occupational health therefore comes as no surprise concerning its state of ambivalence. The progress to promote health is only entertained on a latterly basis where much of the focus and responsibility rests on the individual.

Occupational health services exist in the majority of large manufacturing companies and an increasing number of those in the retail trade provide services also in coal, railways, electricity, gas, steel and dock works. Not all medical services employed have qualifications in occupational medicine and so are concerned mainly with treatment of work injuries, illness and minor ailments occurring at work. It is estimated that 85 per cent of companies employing 34 per cent of the working population provide no service other than statutory first aid cover.

Generally, the services covered by occupational health departments vary depending on their locality. For example, a hospital-based department may provide a service for employers within that hospital and environs. This may also include provisions for the local council and small industries. There are likely to be moves towards provision for primary care groups once they have formed under the *New NHS Modern and Dependable* in April 1999.

For the most part, the components of a standard service includes:

1   identifying and controlling known or suspected hazards and risks to health in the workplace;
2   providing first aid;
3   helping employees with health problems to rehabilitate at work;
4   developing policies to identify and deal with employees problems which might impact on health and safety; and
5   providing information, instruction and training on these matters to employees.

Nine years after the Health and Safety at Work etc., Act 1974 in Britain, occupational health services were still fragmented and unequal. The House of Lords Select Committee on Science and Technology conducted an enquiry under the Chairmanship of Lord Gregson into the future provision of occupational health and hygiene services. The Gregson Report was published in 1983. The report highlighted the rudimentary but extensive services provided by the NHS; small firms had little or no provision. Civil and military services, as well as large manufacturing industry was well catered for.

The extension of occupational health services was considered necessary, especially in medium and smaller enterprises. The Committee attached considerable importance to preventive medicine and pointed out that early detection of hazards at work, and the timely adoption of preventive measures would not alleviate individual suffering, they would lighten the financial burden which sickness imposes on the state. Occupational health was seen as an integral part of the primary care of patients. Again, another call was made for doctors and nurses to be appropriately qualified for the service.

The Gregson Committee concluded that occupational health services should continue to be provided on a private basis founded largely by employers on reflection of their general duty under section II of the Health and Safety at Work etc., Act. Although it recommended an increase in government statutory support, there was reluctance to take such a step for several reasons. Firstly, it would create demand for trained personnel greater than the supply available. Secondly, it would impose an unwelcome and immediate additional cost to industry, so provoking hostility and resentment where co-operation and sympathy was crucial. Finally, it would lead to increased bureaucracy where there was already insufficient flexibility to meet varying needs.

The pressure continued a year later from the Committee who tried to persuade the government of the necessity of services in small and medium enterprises (SME). Gregson warned that a voluntary code was not good enough and legislation was to be the most direct route for achieving their aims.

In the interim period, the ILO established the principle of protecting employees at work in convention 161, 1985. It defined work health and safety services as entrusted with essentially preventive functions and responsibilities for advising the employer, the workers and their representatives on:

- requirements for establishing and maintaining a safe and healthy working environment which will facilitate optimal physical and mental health; and
- the adaptation of work to the capabilities of workers in light of their state of physical and mental health.

These suggestions, it was hoped, would lead to occupational services becoming available for all workers, and that they would be adequate and appropriate to the risks they faced. These services, it was felt, should develop as teams of specialised professionals independent of employers, workers and their representatives.

ILO Convention 161 underlined much of the current thinking on the prevention of ill health in the workforce. However, many employers have made little progress in adopting the strategies enshrined in this convention because successive British governments have never ratified it. Government and employer arguments against doing so relate to the lack of available expertise, and where it exists, the 'prohibitive' cost of buying it. However, the expertise is available if drawn upon and compared to the benefits in human terms – the investment of time, effort and money in the provision of these services is widely held as a small price to pay.

European links

Five years after Gregson, the European Framework Directive on Health and Safety set out its requirements for services. These were designed to prevent ill health at the workplace. In Britain, there was still dependence on the voluntary code. Many employers simply did not understand their specific role in health and safety matters and so provision was left largely to major enterprises and the public sector. For many small firms, full in-house services are an impossible expense. Even on a part time basis, employers think safety advice is costly and so are cautious about drawing on consultancy services. A factory's occupational health department may be no more than an occasional visit by an interested local general practitioner.

The picture has altered in Britain since the incorporation of European legislation into the British health and safety regulations. Following the adoption of the Social Charter in 1989 (Britain did so much later under the Labour government; although health and safety issues were largely adopted at this time), the Commission immediately followed up with a Social Action Programme for its implementation which proposed 47 initiatives. Many of these were legally binding directives which covered the area of industrial relations. The directives relating to health and safety at work were largely adopted. They were subject to a qualified majority voting which could not be vetoed by one member state.

Issues impacting on women were also included under the directives for pregnant women and women recently given birth. The Directive was passed in October 1992 and women became eligible for 14 weeks maternity leave with at least 80 per cent of salary. The UK imposed qualifying conditions for statutory paid maternity leave. An example of this was having to work for the same employer for at least 2 years. This was not in keeping with other member states as maternity leave in many European countries was already quite generous. The final directive conceded a qualifying period of no more than 12 months. The second, more broader outcome of health and safety policy under the Action Programme is the Directive on working time. This Directive was passed in November 1993, and set the minimum daily and weekly rest periods, regulated night and shiftwork, and established a maximum working week of 48 hours. Important concessions to the British government were made including a 7 year implementation period, a dispensation allowing voluntary agreements exceeding the 48 hour week, and exemptions for the fishing, transport and security industries (Ginsburg 1996).

Existing legislation imposes duty on employers to make their workplaces healthy, safe and legal. To do this, employers do require competent advice. The prevention of ill health at work is not uniquely a medical problem. Workers can become ill as a result of exposure to toxic substances, physical agents or negative stress. So when sources of health risk are identified, prevention becomes a matter of seeking advice from the appropriate specialist.

Sources of support: roles and functions

Occupational physicians

Occupational physicians are responsible for advising managers on the identification of an assessment of risk in the workplace. The issue has become a developing phenomenon in the workplace since the late 1980s. It is now a main feature of European legislation whereby managers are duty bound to assess risks within their own environment. It has made for increasing bureaucracy within workplaces but at the same time raised awareness concerning potential hazards.

Occupational physicians are also involved in locating and applying relevant control measures in conjunction with the employer. For example, locating the main source of the problem whether it be chemical, physical or environmental and finding ways of reducing the effects of the problem. This can range from the use of masks to prevent flash burns as a result of welding, to reducing heart problems by encouraging a new system of working for employees. First aid and welfare measures are also extended to the duties of the occupational physician and many are involved in teaching others how to administer basic first aid in the course of their employment.

Their routine work involves health surveillance of workers who may be exposed to hazardous agents including noise, radiation, toxic substances, vibration, biological hazards, physical and psychological stressors. Advice for workers doing jobs which may aggravate an existing condition is part of their duty. They work in collaboration with the individual employee and manager to arrive at suitable accommodation in the event of alternative job placement and rehabilitation as a result of sickness or injury.

Occupational health nurses

Nurses have largely been associated with services to the workplace in Britain since the 1930s. Between 1931 and 1934 special consideration was given to a post basic course for nurses engaged in work in industry. Bedford College for Women and the Royal College of Nursing jointly wrote a course and enrolled one student during the first year. It later became established and was examined by the Royal College of Nursing. This is borne out by the availability of training for registered nurses since 1934 and for enrolled nurses since 1972. Their service provision is various with focus on either being primary health care personnel or as managers or members of a nursing team in medium or large enterprises.

It was the recommendation of the World Health Organization's Expert Committee on Nursing that:

> ... every general probationer and every nurse should have some knowledge of industrial health ... the view was expressed that industrial health should be regarded as an essential part of public health, and that isolated courses of training in the industrial health branch for persons without prior public health training should be discouraged.
>
> Cunningham and Cousens 1953

Their development in the service has been slow, especially during the period 1969 to 1989, a period of intense investigation and political conflict as far as workplace health development was concerned. This is despite the fact that the late 1960s and early 1970s saw a period of full employment and economic prosperity. The majority of occupational health nurses were employed in manufacturing industries such as the motor trade, food, textiles, pharmaceuticals and engineering. Others were employed in large nationalised industries such as British Steel, the National Coal Board, the Post Office, the Water Authorities, British Gas and the Ministry of Defence, as well as the NHS.

The 1980s saw a considerable decline in the patterns of employment, and the majority of nurses were now employed in the service sector, i.e. the NHS and local and central government services. The privatised industries have retained some of their occupational health nurses. Growth in financial, commercial and retail services has seen a move for nurses also in this direction.

Occupational health nurses carry out many of the functions listed under the role of the physician. They have a close relationship with the workforce and are pivotal to the success of surveillance and health education programmes. Given sufficient scope, they are able to provide a permanent focus for occupational health activity in the workplace or in group schemes, where they are able to draw on other sources of expertise in medicine, hygiene and related services as required.

The occupational health service in Britain is about to undergo a serious revision in light of the altering economic scene and the fact that many hazards are better controlled. Public health issues will be encroaching more markedly in occupational health services but this is as yet still under development.

Occupational health nurses, however, continue to be under tremendous strain in terms of professional progress and recognition for the work they undertake. This appears to be for a whole host of reasons, some economic, others political and historic. Firstly, there are a lack of training and education opportunities for many nurses in the UK. There is a poor infrastructure for introductory courses and programmes that specialise in occupational health nursing. Continuing education programmes are fewer, hence reduced ability to gain motivation for updating in this changing field. This problem is allied to the lack of legislation requiring nurses to seek a statutory qualification in this field. Secondly, the government's insistence on a policy of self regulation in health and safety. During times of economic instability, redundancies and the employment of agency staff or cheaper less qualified staff has hampered the development of the profession and the quality of service provision. This is allied to a poor commitment by the government to training which has a knock-on effect in industry where employers will be far more reluctant to provide funding for this development.

The economic benefits of occupational health services are not readily considered by managers. Although such bodies as the CBI and TUC are ready to work in collaboration with employers, occupational health services are frequently considered to be an after thought where active support is not always readily visible when other agendas are involved.

The fifth issue relates to the lack of research into the cost benefits of occupational health services and the necessity of employing occupational health nurses in Britain. Germany, Scandinavia and the US have all entertained such notions with some interesting results. The general message appears that such services are needed but must be qualified with the necessity to account for hidden costs largely found in capital expenditure, e.g. equipment and training. There is also a dearth of research relating to the opinions of those on the receiving end of services who are the missing link in making suggestions for improvement and development. It will be interesting to see if these issues are assessed in the review of the services in Britain.

Occupational hygienist

The role of the occupational hygienist has a long history. For the most part their role related to the prevention of diseases. These included pneumoconiosis, a lung disease often contracted by miners and quarry workers; acute lead poisoning, silicosis in the cutlery industry, bladder cancer produced by dyestuffs and in the rubber industry. Asbestosis was another problem for the occupational hygienist, and although there are now greater controls and measures taken with this substance, the long period of disease development (often between 20 and 50 years) continues to hamper progress in this field.

Today, occupational hygienists provide advice relating to the recognition, evaluation and control of environmental factors in the workplace which may adversely affect the health and comfort of people at work. The factors include: airborne fibres, dusts, gases, micro-organisms and vapours that are likely to be inhaled or absorbed through the skin. Contact with chemicals have been estimated to produce 80,000 cases per year of contact occupational dermatitis in the UK. This can become a disabling condition where prognosis of recovery is often poor. There are in addition, some 500 cases of occupational asthma contracted a year in Britain.

Occupational hygienists are also involved in providing advice and guidance relating to noise/vibration affecting workers' hearing or circulation. Around a million people in Britain are exposed to levels of noise that could damage their hearing. A key requirement of the 1989 Noise at Work Regulations is noise assessment. Employers are encouraged to take action at three levels:

- Where the noise level is at least 85 dba and above 90 dba, a noise assessment is to be undertaken by a trained person. If there have been significant changes in the work environment, such an assessment must be made once every 2 years. Car protectors can be provided by the employer but the employee must take the initiative to request such equipment.
- If noise is above 90 dba then the employer is encouraged to reduce the level of noise as far as is reasonably practicable. Training, instruction and supervision in the wearing of ear protectors in this instance is vital.
- Above 140 dba, known as peak action level where noise is very loud, then the same requirements regarding reduction and protection apply.

Occupational hygienists are also involved in providing guidance to employers on matters relating to ionising and non-ionising radiators, heat or cold and ventilation measures. Ergonomists, engineers and occupational psychologists also form a valuable link in the provision of information, guidance, training, assessment and support services.

Health and safety advisor

Seeking competent health and safety advice is a major issue in the improvement and management of health and safety at work. It is also a legal requirement. Since 1992, under the Management of Health and Safety at Work Regulations, the role of the health and safety advisor has gained prominence. Their role and functions are extensive and include many facets. The purpose is to ensure efficient execution of organisation policy and to monitor employee compliance to regulations. Generally, the role encompasses the following:

- carrying out workplace surveys and risk assessments to assess compliance with health and safety standards;
- investigating the cause of any accidents or dangerous occurrences and recommending means of preventing their occurrence;
- supervising the recording and analysis of information, injuries, ill health, damage and production losses, assessing accident trends and reviewing overall safety performance;
- assisting with training at all levels;

- keeping contact with official and professional bodies such as the Health and Safety Executive (HSE) and Medical Divisions;
- liaison with safety representatives and committees;
- fostering within the workplace, an understanding that injury prevention and damage control are an integral part of business and operational efficiency;
- keeping up to date with recommended codes of practice and new safety literature;
- preparing budgets and obtaining approval for funds to implement policies as related to safety, health and welfare;
- liaison with client's representatives and subcontractors on health and safety issues;
- liaison with employers' insurance companies.

Generally, maintaining health at work involves the coverage of several domains, largely in the interest of the employer. This should not always be the case, but in terms of evolution relating to health and health protection in Britain, legislation and voluntarism has largely undermined the employee position. However, in large measure the service has included the following:

1 *Planning* – the purpose is to achieve early elimination of risk. This enables professionals to fulfil their most important obligations of ill health prevention. This is frequently based on verified information produced by the legal requirements placed on manufacturers relating to research and product information.

2 *Monitoring* – recognizing, monitoring and controlling hazards is an established role in protecting the health of workers. The work includes regular inspection and initial assessment of environmental conditions (noise, dust, thermal conditions, exposure to atmospheric pollutants, contact with chemicals and micro-organisms). It is through monitoring that clinical observation and medical screening of the workforce assume any real relevance.

3 *Health surveillance* – failure to link the results of environmental and clinical monitoring is a major source of weakness in occupational health practice. Sometimes scarce medical resources are devoted to extensive routine medical examinations which can help to detect general health problems for the client who is referred to the NHS. Health surveillance and screening ought to be used as a mechanism for tackling individual health problems and checking the efficacy of established control measures.

4 *Record keeping* – any surveillance undertaken without satisfactory and standardised systems of record keeping is likely to be of limited value in controlling workplace risk. Requirements under COSHH 1995 on the keeping and use of occupational health records and the results of

hygiene monitoring mean that a much more systematic approach needs to be adopted. RIDDOR 1995 also raises persistent problems. Computer technology and adequate support maintenance is considered to be vital.

5   *Research* – health and safety services carry out and support joint research projects in order to assess and monitor health and safety problems in workplaces and industries with similar hazards. Such projects can assist in avoiding duplication of effort and generalise useful experience and lessons gained in specific situations. Trade union involvement is also vital, in advising on appropriate methods, new areas of development, or implementation of screening procedures in the interest of employees. The legal basis for such involvement already exists since the provisions of the SRSCR entitling safety representatives to keep abreast of the results and conduct occupational health research in their place of work.

6   *Fitness for work* – the health examination mechanism provides the employer with suitable information to make an informed decision relating to work demands of employees. Employees who are likely to require alternative work or adjustment in their work regime, or continued medical surveillance, up to the time of full resumption of normal work duties, should have the benefit of an occupational health service.

Confidentiality and mutual trust are important in any discussion between doctor and patient. Disclosure of workers difficulties in coping with their work must not lead to transfer, downgrading or even redundancy. However, employers should arrange for alternative and comparable employment or suitable retraining. Managers and trade union representatives should also be involved in the consultation and decision making process so a mutually beneficial agreement is reached by all parties concerned.

Issues of accountability

The position of any health representative is regarded as ambiguous within the organisation. They may be seen as functionaries of management and therefore do not necessarily have the complete trust of the workforce. Some employers may even regard the company doctor as their employee and expect co-operation in such questions as sickness absence, compensation claims and disclosure of confidential information about individual workers, The occupational health service executes their responsibilities with professional integrity but frequently suffer from isolation and pressures from management.

Their role is one where often channels of communication must be maintained. The mechanisms of accountability and control include the following:

- the appointment or dismissal of occupational health and safety staff should be subject to joint agreement between employers and unions;
- the activities and work programmes of health and safety services should be subject to periodic review and agreement;
- in the case of group services, trade union influence should be exerted through representation at the level of an administrative board;
- targets for the improvement of health and safety should be agreed using appropriate industrial relations procedures;
- safety representatives should have the right to receive regular reports from occupational health and safety personnel to enable them to monitor progress towards these targets;
- trade unionists should also maintain the right to call in or seek advice from either their own or the employer's occupational health staff where necessary. Safety representatives should also be able to assess whether health and safety staff have appropriate training and qualifications.

Recent regulatory developments

Health protection

The Management of Health and Safety at Work Regulations 1992 recognises that the major responsibility for health improvement and protection at work lies with the employer. Particular responsibility is endowed on those providing temporary, contract or short term workers. The regulations outlined below depicts main features relating to risk assessment, health surveillance, the necessity for qualifications and seeking competent help as well as the provision of information and the issues of operating on multiple sites.

Risk assessment

Assessing risk places the onus of responsibility on the employer to minimise health problems and accidents at the workplace. Risk at work, is perceived in terms of hazard or potential hazard and its likely impact on the worker as well as the company. A hazard is a phenomenon that is likely to lead to, or cause harm if not dealt with in the appropriate manner (Table 1). The hazard in regulation relates largely to the environment, occupation of space, time and mechanics. Rarely do they relate to the individual except in cases of competence to perform a specific task. The notion of competence connects with the expectation that the individual has been trained, is able to apply their new found knowledge and skill in an appropriate way, as well as knowledge of their limitations. Regulation 3 states: Undoubtedly, this is an area that requires further exploration in an era where there are increasing

Table I   Steps in assessing risk

1   Identify hazards
2   Reduce to a minimum or eliminate hazards
3   Evaluate the remaining risks
4   Develop strategies
5   Provide training for those involved in new work procedures and methods
6   Implement precautionary measures
7   Monitor procedure and performance
8   Review and modify periodically

employers are required to:
- carry out risk assessment of any work activities that may put anyone at risk;
- take particular account of the inexperience of young persons, and risks to women who are of child-bearing age, pregnant or nursing mothers, from working methods and the use of chemicals;
- use the assessment to determine the precautions necessary to protect against the identified hazards. The precautionary measures to overcome or reduce the hazards identified will depend on the work circumstances;
- repeat the assessment if the work changes;
- record the assessment if there are more than five employees.

numbers of cases reported relating to harassment, usually in the form of bullying or subtle sexisms and racism in terms of verbalistic expression and the use of language to undermine the individual rather than support them in their work and development. Indeed bullying is a major occupational health problem costing employers £5 billion a year and up to 6 million working days lost (Guardian, Jan 1999). The harassment comes as a product along a continuum of frustration, bitching and anger at circumstances in which certain employees find themselves. Managers are also often found to be the perpetrators of such behaviour (Pringle 1988; Guardian 1999).

Assessing such risks are shot full of potential problems as they enter the domain of the personal as opposed to the professional. Naturally, one expects people to behave in a professional manner in the work environment. However, with many powerful forces operating agendas for goods and services, then the politicking which is usually quite an aberration of incorrectness that the unravelling of such issues can be lost in poor procedures and policies in the workplace. A workplace is more likely to protect those who are the perpetrators of psychological violence rather than its victims to save public face. Risk assessment is an inexact science because it is based on subjective criteria of what presents a risk. One person's perceptions and standards differ from another.

Health surveillance

This is usually carried out by a person with expertise in the field of monitoring disease and illness at work. The fact that surveillance has come to mean a form of checking in the whole evidence based phenomena, and its trails of hazards and health problems is no mistake. In an age of target setting, consciousness about health problems, greater availability of information means that such surveillance cannot be avoided. Regulation 5 states:

health surveillance is to be provided to employees where an occupational disease or health risk is identified:* if an identifiable disease or health risk is likely under normal foreseeable work conditions;* carried out by a suitably qualified person, i.e. occupational health nurse or doctor.

The use of technology can tell us at the touch of a button, the health problems of the organisation within a given period of time. Such information can be utilised in a positive way to determine programmes, policies and strategies for dealing with potential/actual health problems at work. It can be a positive link for health promoters and occupational health staff in terms of collaborative working for the benefit of the individual and the organisation. The company can also more accurately predict the likelihood of health problems and adapt its systems and work patterns to enable this process to operate smoothly. However, this is not always the case in the teeth of the necessity for increased productivity, or in keeping pace with change that is internal and influenced by the external, for example, political climate or economic downturns. Joined up thinking is required in organisations to maximise the reduction in hazards and to improve health.

Health surveillance for the worker operates in terms of provision of information and symptoms to the health practitioner to enable him or her to make a diagnosis. If any treatment is required then this is recorded and such documentation is kept for up to 40 years.

Regulation 11

Health Surveillance is to be carried out by the employment medical adviser or appointed doctor, every 12 months where an employee works in specified processes with:

- vinyl chloride monomer
- nitro or amino derivatives of phenol and benzene
- potassium or sodium chromate or dichromate
- 1-naphthylamine and its salts
- dianisidine and its salts
- dichlorobenzidine and its salts
- auramine; magenta; carbon disulphide
- disulphur dichlodride
- benzene and benzol
- carbon tetrachloride
- trichlorethylene
- pitch

where exposure occurs to any other hazardous substance which could give rise to an identifiable ill health condition. Records of health surveillance to be kept for 40 years. If the medical adviser bars an employee from working with a particular substance the employer must ensure this happens. Medical examinations should take place during normal working hours. Employees must be allowed to see their medical records. The Medical Adviser may inspect the work place if she/he wishes. Appeals against a medical decision must be made to the Health and Safety Executive.

Qualifications and competent help

The Regulations identify the necessity for health improvement and protection in the workplace to be structured and well informed. There are a range of competences that can be demonstrated:

1 *Full time health and safety consultant* – such persons are qualified in health and safety having a university degree in occupational health and safety or having passed part II of the NEBOSH Diploma examination or its NVQ level 4 equivalent. In addition, they must possess a number of years practical experience in the field, or be a member of IOSH with a Registered Safety Practitioner (RSP) certificate, or registered MIIRSM with the British Safety Council (BSC).

2 *Part time appointees* – the necessity for such expertise is dependent on the type of risk that exists within the organisation.

   - high risk: degree or at least part I NEBOSH Diploma; practical experience,

- lesser risk: NEBOSH National General Certificate; familiarity with work area,
- low risk: NEBOSH National General Certificate; IOSH 'Managing Safely' certificate; familiarity with work area.

3 *Professional consultancy* – a necessary degree of knowledge and expertise in the field is expected, and the employer is to provide sufficient resources to enable the expert to convey an appropriate level of advice.

Provision of information

Regulation 8 states that:

all employees are to be provided with comprehensible and relevant information on:-the risks they face in their work including any that result from multi-occupancy of the premises;- precautions and preventative measures in place to protect them;- emergency procedures and who the emergency marshals are;- where a child is employed the parents must be given the above information.

The provision or at least awareness of sources information within the organisation is crucial to ensure health improvement and health protection for all. These may come in the source of legal procedures and documents or publications from the HSE, Health Education Authority and their equivalents in Scotland, Wales and Northern Ireland, or bodies with an interest in employee protection ROSPA, or Health Alliance groups.

Multiple sites

Working or having operations on multiple sites creates problems in terms of communication and maintaining consistency of service. The Regulation makes clear how this issue should be negotiated:

Where two or more employers share the same premises (multi-occupancy):- they must co-operate in meeting statutory obligations;- they must keep each other informed of specific risks arising from their particular operations;- these obligations may be met by appointing a safety co-ordinator for the premises;- where self-employed persons share premises they too must co-operate for the common good;- where someone other than the employer has control over part of the work premises (i.e. a landlord), he too must co-operate with his tenant employers to ensure health and safety in the various workplaces. This is in addition to any responsibility he carries for common areas under his direct control, i.e. entrance halls, stairs, lifts, etc.

The health and safety executive

The Health and Safety Executive (HSE) have an interest in the health and safety of people at work. This includes people who may be harmed by the way work is done (for example because they live near a factory, or are passengers on a train). In some situations, they are also concerned with the way work affects the environment.

The HSE is involved with inspection as well as developing health and safety laws, codes and standards which cover safe working right across industry, publish advice and guidance and carry out research. They also play a full part in international developments, especially in the European Union. They have a close working relationship with employers, trade unions and experts in many fields, and occasionally draw upon employers to provide assistance.

The HSE covers factories, building sites, mines, farms, fairgrounds, quarries, railways, chemical plant, offshore and nuclear installations, schools and hospitals. It tends to be local authority officers who tend to cover retailing, some warehouses, offices, hotels and catering, sports, leisure, consumer services and places of worship.

Officers are involved with enforcing laws including:

- the Health and Safety at Work etc., Act 1974
- COSHH Regulations and the Workplace (Health, Safety and Welfare) Regulations 1994
- laws covering hazards, e.g., Food and Environment Protection Act and Control of Pesticides Regulations
- laws which pre-date the HASWA, e.g. a range of factories acts
- laws covering nuclear industry, mining, railway, explosives, offshore oil, and gas industries.

Other services are listed in Table 2.

Health improvement

In February 1998, the Labour government published its Green Paper on Public Health which identified the workplace as one of three key settings for action – along with schools and neighbourhoods – to reduce preventable death in four major areas:

- heart disease and stroke, of which 25,000 die each year
- accidents
- cancer, where 32,000 die each year
- mental health

It was specifically designed to outline the government's plans for health improvement across the population and to develop a strategy to reduce inequalities.

Table 2   Other services

Sharing services	This option has not been developed to any significant extent but is one possibility. For example, subcontractors can be required within contract conditions to use a main contractor's OH services or provide equivalent cover from other sources. There is also scope for exploring ways of sharing the services of safety officers and safety reps to provide basic health and safety assessment and advice in workplaces within the same industry or locality, or along a company's supply chain.
Group safety schemes	These are concentrated mainly in the construction industry and involve sharing the services of a qualified safety officer between a number of employers usually involved in the same industry.
NHS services	There are a limited number of consultants in the NHS in occupational medicine and a limited number of general practitioners with qualifications in occupational health. Some hospitals offer occupational health and safety services to 'clients' on a fee generating basis.
Consultancy	There are a wide variety of organisations offering medical, safety and hygiene services to employers. Some are relatively small and are sometimes based on individual specialists. Some are larger organisations operating on a fee for service basis. A number are based in university departments. Wherever such services are used, it is important to assess their professional competence and past record.
Employers' and trade associations	A number of trade associations provide health and safety services and advice to member companies. These can vary from specialist medical and scientific services to general information and guidance on common hazards in specific sectors.
Joint Industry Scheme	In a number of areas, for example agriculture and the rubber industry, the TUC has proposed jointly controlled schemes under HSC Industry Advisory Committees. These would cover particular industry sectors and act as clearing houses for health and safety service needs and promote and co-ordinate health and safety service activity, sharing information and research findings wherever possible.

For the first time in almost 20 years, the social situations that contribute to poor health were exposed openly by the government. This is against the backdrop of the drive to increase efficiency in health care, curtail the perceived excessive expenditure on public services and enhance quality in health care. Research into inequalities in health began to gain pace during the 1980s prompted by the Black Report (Black et al. 1980), the WHO's Health For All by the Year 2000 and Healthy Public Policy initiatives (WHO 1981, 1988), and the 'New Public Health' movement in Britain which openly endorsed anti-poverty measures. This was largely ignored by the Tory government. *Our Healthier Nation* sets the scene for environmental and public health, as well as an agenda for health promotion. However, it must be noted that it is only a framework and hence it is for health service, environmental health and safety, and public health and other service workers and users to make their contribution to achieving better health. Developments will be publicised later this year.

Although the statutory requirement to provide workplace health and safety services – as outlined in ILO Convention 161 – is no closer, and the voluntary codes still holds sway under this new development, the spirit of social partnership is encouraged. The Government commits itself to setting standards of health and safety in the environment and supporting the HSE's *Good Health is Good Business* campaign. With the Health and Safety Commission, the government is drawing up plans for a 10 year strategy for occupational health.

However, it expects that employers could also commit by:

- having excellent standards of health and safety management;
- taking measures to reduce stress at work;
- creating flexible working arrangements bearing in mind employee's home lives and child care responsibilities;
- ensuring a smoke free working environment;
- contributing to and implementing the '10 year strategy';
- making healthy choices (healthy canteens and cycle stores) easy for staff.

The third social partner in this new arrangement is the employee. They, the government hopes, will commit to:

- following health and safety rules and guidelines;
- working directly or through safety reps to create a healthy working environment;
- supporting colleagues with problems or disabilities;
- contributing to charitable and social work through work based voluntary organisations.

The effect of health on work is a legitimate concern for all involved in health protection and health improvement. However, increasingly, time should be spent on health promotion, which uses the workplace as a contact point for more general public services. The Labour government argues:

Being in work is good for health. Joblessness has been clearly linked to poor physical and mental health. Unemployed men and women are more likely than people in work to die from cancer, heart disease, accidents and suicide. Losing his job doubles the chances of a middle-aged man dying within the next 5 years.

Department of Health 1998

The Government recognises that the social causes of ill health and the inequalities which stem from them must be acknowledged and acted on. Indeed they state:

Connected problems require joined up solutions. This means tackling inequality which stems from poverty, poor housing, pollution, low educational standards, joblessness and low pay. Tackling inequalities generally is the best means of tackling health inequalities in particular.

Department of Health 1998

With reference to the workplace, this source of inequality rests with poor practices, lack of training and adequate skills to carry out the task required of employees in a rapidly changing environment, as well as inadequate financial reward. The health movement cannot directly account for the inequity in pay, but it can persuade employers that maintaining a satisfactory work environment can protect, improve and maintain health. Indeed, part of the government's economic case has underlined this point:

To succeed in the modern world economy, the country's workforce must be healthy as well as highly skilled. The Confederation of British Industry has estimated that 187 million working days are lost each year because of sickness. That's a £12 billion social tax on business every year. This can damage a company's competitiveness and put a brake on prosperity.

Department of Health 1998

With specific relevance to disease they argue:

Cancer treatments cost the NHS an estimated £1.3 billion each year, whilst heart disease, stroke and related illnesses costs some £1.2 billion, and treating poor mental health in excess of £5 billion a year. Illnesses caused by smoking cost the NHS between £1.4 and £1.7 billion each year. By preventing avoidable illnesses, the NHS can concentrate its resources on treating those conditions which cannot yet be prevented.

Department of Health 1998

Table 3 The contract for health

Government and national players	Local players and communities	People
Provide national co-ordination and leadership	Provide leadership for local health strategies by developing and implementing health improvement programmes.	Take responsibility for their own health and make healthier choices about their lifestyle
Ensure that policy making across government takes full account of health and is well informed by research and the best expertise available	Work in partnerships to improve the health of local people and tackle the root causes of ill health	Ensure their own actions do not harm the health of others
Work with other countries for international co-operation to improve health.	Plan and provide high quality services to everyone who needs them.	Take opportunities to better their lives and their families lives, through education, training and employment.
Assess risks and communicate those risks clearly to the public Ensure that the public and others have the information they need to improve their health Regulate and legislate where necessary Tackle the root causes of ill health		

The contract for health

To bring the nation together in a concerted and co-ordinated drive against poor health, the government proposes a national contract for the better. The contract sets out mutual responsibilities of employers, employees and other interested parties for improving health in the areas where the most progress can be made towards the overall aims of reducing the numbers of early deaths, increasing the length of healthy lives and tackling inequalities in health (Table 3).

The government identifies two key aims:

- to improve the health of the population as a whole by increasing the length of people's lives and the number of years people spend free from illness;

- to improve the health of the worst off in society and to narrow the health gap.

Priority areas

The government has focussed on the following areas to seek health improvement in the form of targets.

By the Year 2010:

- heart disease and stroke – to reduce the death rate from heart disease and stroke and related illnesses amongst people aged under 65 years by at least a further third;
- accidents – to reduce accidents by at least a fifth;
- cancer – to reduce the death rate from cancer amongst people aged under 65 years by a further fifth;
- mental health – to reduce the death rate from suicide and undetermined injury by at least a further sixth.

The workplace is one of the priority areas for action in terms of health improvement. The patchy history towards achieving health in the work environment has brought us closer to the issues and problems that exist. The next chapter provides an interrogation of work and the organisation and its impact on the individual.

Chapter 4

The work, the organisation and the individual

This chapter discusses the issue of work and the peculiarity of the work process, and how they impinge upon individual workers. A connection with the health problems which develop as a result of work organisation and working relationships is demonstrated.

Nature and purpose

The purpose and nature of work has an evolutionary history. Work is largely performed for gain, whether it be to obtain produce from the land as mere self subsistence or for monetary gain by way of sale for profit. Work can also be pleasure as it is borne out of the need to be active and to engage in something useful to extend knowledge, provide for a family or care for others. Work is a necessity of life, and yet, it is performed in the most diverse ways to achieve the universally necessary goal providing the sustenance of life. Recognizing this diversity leads to admiration for human ingenuity, endurance and skill.

During the 6th century AD, new ideas concerning the meaning of work were introduced. However, these were largely confined to members of monastic brotherhoods and tended to lose their force as monastic orders became increasingly powerful. The idea of work as ennobling began to pass from the monastic orders to new men in the late Middle Ages – merchants, artisans and traders who wanted to find merit in their own pursuits (Neff 1968).

Work perceived as the satisfaction of human needs, can be a problem. It encourages the notion that humans can sanction the use of the natural world for their own needs. It contains the danger that such an idea sees the natural world as exploitable rather than as an aid to human endeavour to be used with care. Some Eastern philosophies such as Buddhism regard work was having little special meaning only in relation to one's philosophy of life and in harmonizing the being of the individual with the totality of nature. Buddha teaches that '... If work is to have the best of meanings it must contribute to decreasing misery, grief, anguish or pain' (Sui 1971).

Work was regarded as a path to salvation and had its origins in religious controversies. Enthusiastic traders, merchants and artisans as supporters of Protestant reforms communicated that work should be seen as a path to individual salvation. This position was again popularised in the nineteenth century and influenced the works of Durkheim and Weber.

Although 'work' was increasingly seen as 'good', the rapidly developing division of labour in the manufacturing society up to the 1970s in the industrialised world, generated additional subtleties of meaning. Distinctions arose between mental and manual labour, between the skilled and unskilled, and between the labour of the manager and the labour of the hands.

The differentiation of work came about as a result of the evolution into an agricultural and pastoral society. This differentiation became more apparent with the expansion of agriculture and the institution of slavery. It was later that the distinction between 'labour' and 'work' was developed. Arendt used the term 'animal laborens' to describe the kind of work which repetitiously produced the essential consumable goods necessary for the maintenance of life. She also used the term 'homo faber' for the production of craftsmen or artisans. At a higher level, the Greeks and Romans devoted their labour in politics, war and the management of human relations. Some of these notions formed the foundations of the modern workplace.

Work became differentiated between skilled and unskilled, productive and non-productive, blue collar, white collar and professional, waged work and voluntary work. There have also been divisions of work associated with different historical eras, namely: primary-extractive and agricultural work associated with the pre-industrial period; secondary manufacturing and factory work associated with the industrial period; tertiary, services and information associated with the modern, computer and post-industrial age; and the predicted quaternary of leisure activities and voluntary work associated with societies in the twenty-first century. The pace of change in terms of work activity in the run up to the twenty-first century, however, has depicted new forms of work linked less with leisure and more with knowledge and service and less with human interaction.

Defining work

Attempts have been made over the generations to gather empirical evidence on the definition of work: Freidmann and Havighurst (1954) used interviews and questionnaires among steel workers, sales people, miners, printers and physicians. The approaches aimed to ascertain the meaning of work for each occupational group. Those considered in the skilled/manual category, defined work as *making a living*. The Kahn and Weiss (1960) study pursued the difference between work and non-work and found that work was perceived to be a necessary evil and something for which they were paid. By contrast, non-work was seen as something to be enjoyed.

Margione (1973) made a categorical distinction between work, job and occupation. Subjects were asked to attach meanings to these terms. Both *work* and *occupation* were characterised by one definition: 'Work' was *not enjoyed* and 'occupation' was *something an individual was paid for*. More recent uses of the word occupation is to identify work activities. It is a fundamental term describing what people do to earn a living, emphasising that it is work which sustains life. Thus, work includes both making things and performing services which are of value to oneself, as well as to others. *Job* on the other hand was not clearly characterised by a single definition but rather combined elements of displeasure, remuneration and requirement. Work was seen as a means of survival, a way of obtaining goods and services, and exploiting others.

There is no entirely satisfactory definition of work. This is because it relates to many human activities. Work has been defined as making things and at the same time, has been related to needs. However, making things and utilitarian work are not the only types of work. There are also people who provide services in the sense of teaching, policing and nursing. The forms of work have evolved largely through necessity through the ages and more recently as an adaptation to the capitalist environment and issues connected to globalisation. The process of evolution varies between countries and continents. Politics, economics, geography and socialisation has contributed to the pace of evolution.

Marx's perspective (1818–1883)

Work has also been regarded as a means to salvation, but overall has largely negative connotations. The most developed theoretical explanations regarding the nature of work come from Marx and his followers. The influence has spanned the generations and is still relevant today in terms of a theoretical starting point in the analysis of work, industry and organisation. Marx defined work as the production of goods and services. Work held the key to human happiness and fulfilment. The relations of production are the social relationships associated with the means of production. In a capitalist economy, the relationship of the two main groups in society to the means of production differs sharply – workers simply own their labour which as wage earners they offer for hire to capitalists.

Marx argued that the nature of work in society could be understood by examining its infrastructure. He believed that a capitalist infrastructure inevitably produced a high level of alienation in workers. Like their products, workers are reduced to the level of a commodity. A monetary value is placed on their work and the costs of labour are assessed in the same way as the costs of machinery and raw materials. Like the commodities they manufacture, workers are at the mercy of market forces and the law of supply and demand. Writing and observing conditions in nineteenth century Europe, Marx saw two important characteristics of industrial society: (1)

the mechanisation of production; and (2) the further specialisation of the division of labour.

Both contribute to worker alienation. Marx stressed the capitalist economic system rather than industrialisation as the primary source of alienation. The concept briefly culminates in the individual worker having little control over the goods and services produced, the decision making process over the work performed and distribution of the product. At the same time social relationships between worker and employer are constrained and largely adapt to the forces of capitalism rather than that of nature. Eventually workers estrangement becomes commonplace in home as well as work situations (Giddens 1988). This view became increasingly prominent in the late twentieth century studies of worker health, particularly mental health and stress (Ollman 1971; Eyer 1975, 1977; Eyer and Sterling 1977; Navarro 1976; Garfield 1978, 1979, 1980; Coburn 1979).

Marxist studies on occupational health emphasise the contradictions between profitability and improved health conditions in capitalist industries. Specific research using the Marxist concept of alienation, has clarified the illness generating conditions of the workplace and profit system with reference to disease entities such as asbestos and mesothelioma, complications of vinyl chloride, drug abuse and accidents (Sterner 1943; Patty 1962; Viola et al. 1971; Makk et al. 1974; OSHA 1974; Selikoff and Culyer 1975; Roberts 1977; Cohen 1980; see also Navarro and Gardell, Chapter 5).

Marx explains further that the mechanisation of production reduced the physical effort involved in work but the 'lightening of the labour even becomes a sort of torture. As the machine does not free the labourer from work, but deprives him of all interest' (Pearlin 1981). Mechanisation and associated mass production, particularly dominant until the late 1970s, reduced the need for skill and intelligence, and removed from work all individual character and consequently all charm for the workers. Marx saw individuals as having an exclusive sphere of activity from which they cannot escape. Freedom and fulfilment are not possible when people are imprisoned in a specialised occupation since only a limited part of themselves could be expressed in one job (Rotter 1966).

Later works, in the neo-marxist framework (Gorz 1965; Marcuse 1972), place emphasis on alienation with reference to the consumption of products. According to Gorz, alienation at work leads the worker to seek fulfilment in leisure. However, just as the capitalist system shapes the working day, it also shapes leisure activities. It creates the passive consumer who finds satisfaction in the consumption of products of the manufacturing and entertainment industries.

Leisure simply provides a means of escape and oblivion, a means of living with the problem rather than an active solution to it. Gorz notes that people in a capitalist society are alienated from both work and leisure. The two spheres of life reinforce each other in the process of alienation. From a work and health perspective, Eyer and Karasek (1979, 1984) support Gorz in noting that the social organisation of society and work reinforces symptoms of physical and psychological stress for the worker. Excessive alcohol consumption and other forms of substance abuse including smoking can also be seen as a feature of alienation. The pleasure seeking behaviours outside the work environment is a mechanism for coping with the circumstances (Argyropoulos-Grisanos and Hawkins 1983; Beaumont and Allsop 1983; Webb et al. 1994).

Marcuse's (1972) observations on the same theme saw that potential for personal development is crushed in advanced industrial society. Work is exhausting, stupefying, inhuman slavery. Leisure is based on needs that are false and largely imposed by the mass media controlled by the capitalist forces. Others, including C. Wright Mills (1951), suggested that individuals are alienated at work from their true selves because in the work situation they need to act sincerely and generously in order to manipulate others so they can earn a living.

Work has also been associated with the process of control of managers over workers (Braverman 1974; Bowles and Gintis 1976; Freidmann 1977; Navarro 1988) This is understood by means of:

1   the compartmentalisation of work tasks;
2   hierarchised division of labour reproducing the class relations in society; and
3   people being expropriated from all possibility of controlling, influencing or having a say in the design or development of the work process or of the products they create (see Chapter 1).

Work, under the Marxist notion of alienation, has also been associated with the reproduction of society and its social phenomena. Palloix (1980) notes that it is the mode of organisation of production and the process of work where the roots of the division of social classes are to be found (see Chapter 1). Work, too is associated with the construction of one's personality. Gardell (1987) concluded that unless these needs are satisfied at the workplace, the individual experiences a basic frustration that manifests itself in different efforts to achieve adjustment. This view is also shared by Friedlander (1967) and Gustavsen (1980).

Privatised workers as they were called, were the impetus of consumer society and the emphasis on provision of family needs created a context where workers' commitment centred on the instrumental regularity of the pay packet, regardless of the limits of work satisfaction (Dubin 1956; Ingham 1967; Herzberg 1968; Cotgrove 1972; Wedderburn and Crompton 1972; Gallie 1978).

Seeing the worker as a consumer explains the abundance of studies aimed at understanding the health of individuals by looking at their diet, consumption, levels of expectation, lifestyles, utilisation of health services and residential patterns (COMA 1983). Consequently, the consumer becomes involved in the strategy of social intervention primarily aimed at monetary compensation for the damage created at work. Health is sold to the consumer, and disease and death are compensated.

Criticisms

The Marxist view of alienation was severely criticised by Goldthorpe and Lockwood for not being directly a sociological concept, and as untenable ideological rhetoric limited by a narrow concern with the nature of work. However, Goldthorpe and Lockwood's study (1975) contains no examination of the objective structures of work, and work experience is merely assumed to be understood through survey responses. As Burawoy (1979) notes, there is no distinction made 'between coming to work on the one hand, and working on the other – that is, between the delivery of power and that of labour power'. This view is supported by Martin and Fryer (1975).

Emile Durheim (1858–1917)

What happens on the shop floor and in the work environment is of great importance in developing an understanding of the nature of work (Beynon 1973; Bulmer 1975). Perspectives have been offered by Durkheim concerning the division of labour. Work provides the framework for the production of social solidarity and co-operation. The idea that workplace organisation could be based on a *web of roles* and consensus of values has influenced contemporary sociology. Durkheim recognised that excessive specialisation could result in a disruptive loss of meaning, *anomie*. This has some resonance with the ideas of Marx, however, the impact is more horizontal than hierarchical. Human relations theory noted the varieties of lack of attachment of workers to the organisation and like Durkheim, asserted that a sense of belonging and function be created by altering work group values and managerial skills. However, in contrast to the concept of alienation, anomie fails to recognise the fragmentation of work and hierarchical control that are objective features of the capitalist organisation of production.

Durkheim believed that the specialised division of labour and the rapid expansion of industrial society contained threats to social solidarity. From an economic perspective, this refers to the process of dividing labour into separate and specialised operations with the purpose of increasing production. In a sociological sense, it means the principle of social cohesion which develops in societies whose social bonds result from the way individuals relate when their occupational functions are separate and specialised. This position facilitates the rise of social institutions and social bonds by contract as opposed to sentiment.

The division of labour tended to produce the situation of *anomie* which actually means normlessness. Anomie is present when social controls are weak, when the moral obligations which constrain individuals and regulate their behaviour are not strong enough to function effectively. Durkheim saw a number of indications of anomie in late nineteenth century industrial society, in particular high rates of suicide, marital break up and industrial conflict. Such behaviour indicates a breakdown of normative control.

Industrial society tended to produce anomie for the following reasons. It is characterised by rapid social change which disrupts the norms governing behaviour. In Durkheim's view, the customary limits to what people want and expect from life are disrupted in times of rapid change. Only when desires and expectations are limited by general agreement can people be happy, since unlimited desires can never be satisfied.

In industrial society people became restless and dissatisfied since the traditional ceiling on their desires had largely disintegrated. Increasing prosperity resulting from economic expansion made the situation more acute. A new moral consensus about what people could reasonably expect from life was required. This would involve the regulation of competition in the exchange of goods and services. Exchange must be governed by norms regulating prices and wages which involve the general consensus on issues such as a fair and reasonable return for services. This agreement will set limits on people's desires and expectations.

Not only will rapid social change, but the specialised division of labour itself, tend to produce anomie. It generally encourages individualism and self interest since it is based on individual differences rather than similarities. There is a tendency for the individual to direct his or her own behaviour rather than be guided and disciplined by shared norms. Although Durkheim welcomed this emphasis on individual freedom, he saw it as a threat to social unity. Translated in more modern context, it can be noted that anomie was indeed marked out in many organisations with a change in structure, increased competitiveness, downsizing and short termism, characteristic of the 1980s. It has tended to erode a sense of duty and responsibility towards others, factors which Durkheim saw as essential for social solidarity, but a contributory factor in stress and its related problems.

Arendt's perspective (1906–1975)

Arendt's most important contribution was to differentiate between work and labour. It is comparable to Marx's differentiation between the qualitative aspects of labour and the quantitative aspects of labour. Arendt sees labouring as the undifferentiated use of the body to perform work (qualitative), while work is the use of the hands and head to create man made things which are durable and can be used to create other things. Labouring leads to permanence of substances which are durable.

Arendt (1958) categorises work as part of what she considers to be the three fundamental human activities – labour, work and action. She defines *labour* as corresponding to the biological process of the human body, whose growth, metabolism and eventual decay are part of the life process fed by labour. Life itself is the human condition of labour. *Work* is defined as the activity which corresponds to the artifice of human existence. It is embedded in the ever recurring life cycle. Work provides an artificial world which is distinct from nature. The phenomena created by work defines and transcends the man made world. The human condition of work is the creation of the world in which human beings live and are housed. *Action* is activity not mediated by things or matter. Arendt goes on to communicate the place of work and its connectedness upon the character of human existence:

> Labour assures individual survival. Work bestows permanence and durability from upon mortal life and the fleeting character of human time. Action preserves political bodies and creates the condition for remembrance – that is, for history. The world in which the active life spends itself consists of the man made world of things, which conditions the life of man. No matter what their actions, humans are conditioned beings. Because human existence is conditioned existence, it would be impossible without things, and things would be a heap of unrelated articles, if they were not the conditioners of human existence.
>
> Arendt 1958, pp. 7–8

For Arendt, labouring is a process. It is an endless cycle analogous to the biological processes of a living organism. The end result is death. The cycle is sustained through consumption, and activity which provides the means of consumption is labouring.

Work, however, is different. Work does not prepare matter for incorporation, but changes it into material in order to work upon it and use the finished product. From this standpoint, it is work, as opposed to labour, that is destructive, since the work process takes matter out of the hands of nature without any recompense. Nature does eventually invade the products of work, threatening the durability of the human world. The protection and preservation of the man made world against the natural process – rust, water, wind, heat, cold, earthquakes, floods and more – are among the toils which need the monotonous performance of daily repeated tasks. This is man's struggle through work by which he defends against nature, his durable works, building and monuments, as compared with labour which serves to satisfy his bodily needs and is part of the cycle of nature.

Arendt's position on the limitation of Marx

In applying Arendt's concepts of architecture and the status of objects, there appears an emerging critique of Marx. Arendt's notion of the victory of animal laborens over homo faber – labour over work in the modern world (Frampton 1979). Writing before mass communication rapidly developed, Marx predicted the eventual liberation of mankind from the necessity of the remorseless labour. He did not account for the latent potential of machine production to promote a voracious consumer society 'where nearly all human labour power is spent in consuming with the concomitant serious social problem of leisure' (Arendt 1958, pp. 117–118). Marx could also not foresee that the reduction in working hours would be compensated by the hours wasted in the consumption of means of travel, mainly automobiles, merely to get to work. Arendt points out that, while Marx saw the essence of man as a working animal, animal laborens, he postulated a society in which he foresaw that socialised men would spend their freedom from labouring in those strictly private and essentially worldless activities that we now call hobbies (Arendt 1958). However, this is not so much a contradiction as Arendt believed if we realise that Marx was talking about a society in which people would work voluntarily according to their desires and abilities, rather than having to work from necessity.

Division of labour

Arendt stresses the difference between specialisation and the division of labour. What they have in common is the principle of organisation, which has nothing to do with work or labour but is based on the political sphere of life, the capacity for people to act together in concert. Specialisation of work requires different skills which are pooled. Division of labour adds to labour power. The singularity of division of labour is the opposite of the multiplicity of skills in specialisation of labour. Increasingly, in factory organisation work, labour is homogenised, and the end in view is no longer the product. However, workers gain their subsistence from their labour, nothing else.

Human relations

Arendt had little confidence in the human relations movement in industry, which she saw as an attempt to replace satisfaction that comes from work and craftsmanship, with respect earned by workers from their fellow workers. For her, the slogan *humanism of labour* is a contradiction, because labour, as such, implies a degradation from the craftsmanship of work and from the satisfaction of fabrication. It is the use of bodily labour divorced from the mental and manual powers of creative work.

Summary of Arendt's work

For Arendt, labour is a biological necessity through which people produce things they consume and must produce again. The cycle of production and consumption goes on with rhythmic regularity as long as human life is sustained. Labour produces nothing permanent. It is necessary and futile, necessary for life and futile because it leaves nothing permanent to show. This separates the notion from creativity, ideas and craftsmanship.

Work creates a home for man and protects him from the destructions of nature. It also creates the framework for the social environment and creates conditions for human community. Arendt's distinction between work and labour broadly corresponds to Marx's distinction between concrete and abstract labour.

Work

- Products of work to be used
- Work distinguishes people from their product
- Gives natural material a new shape or form
- Produces objects which stand over against man and enjoy a measure of independence
- Work things are public and objective entities, and are subject to aesthetic considerations
- Reveals craftsmanship in action unique being

Labour

- Products of labour to be consumed
- Assimilates man to nature
- Is mechanical and cyclical in which man adjusts and adapts to the rhythm of processes outside himself such as a machine
- Man accepts external nature
- Labour undertaken to serve human needs is judged by subjective criteria of human desire
- Man reveals his bodily needs through labour

Work is necessary for human existence and assists individuals in creation. This is revealed through the process of work. The action, labour provides exercise, drive and stimulus to enable the fulfilment of human needs.

Conclusion

1   Work and labour reveal what man is. The notions inextricably link to inform personality

2   Action reveals who man is
3   Activities of labour, work and action collectively constitute the world of human praxis, each is indispensable

Fredrick Winslow Taylor (1856–1917)

Taylor published *The Principles of Scientific Management* in 1911 which extended work previously carried out in the field. His main ideas were as follows:

1   Taylor saw workers as individuals with distinct capacities for different types of work and urged that workers' jobs should match their intellect and capabilities. Workers were encouraged to maximise output;
2   he advanced the claim that managerial authority rested on expertise rather than on property rights. Obtaining group harmony through group action was seen as a way forward;
3   the major problem of low productivity at work was the sole responsibility of management and was a result of their ignorance of work process which allowed workers to control the speed and process of work. By acquiring knowledge of the labour process, and simultaneously stripping as many jobs as possible of their skilled content by expanding the division of labour wherever possible, management would regain control and through scientific work study techniques, secure major productivity gains. These could then be shared by the workforce – though their incentive schemes would have to be individually based to deter collective action in the form of unions.

Criticisms

1   Taylor's diagnosis of the industrial situation was based on a simple theme of inefficiency (Rose 1978). Taylor selected the best workers for his experiments and assumed that workers who were not good at one particular task would be best at some other task. There is a lack of certainty here. Taylor implied there was one best way of performing a task which undermined his idea of working with the capabilities of each individual worker.
2   The notion of a fair day's work for a fair day's pay, is not purely a technical matter. It is also a notion of social equity and not in keeping with a scientific approach. There is the suggestion that Taylor's work was misunderstood (Drucker 1981). For Drucker, the central theme of Taylor's work was the need to substitute industrial warfare by industrial harmony. Taylor sought to do this through higher wages from increased output, the removal of physical strain from doing work the wrong way,

development of the workers and the opportunity for them to undertake tasks they were capable of doing. Also the elimination of authoritarian management and an emphasis on guidance for the worker (Mullins 1994).

The Taylorist notion was further developed by Gantt, Munsterberg, Emerson and Fayol. Gantt was the first to introduce the notion of humanism in organisational analysis. He was concerned to boost worker morale through the provision of training to develop their skills in the workplace and financial incentives. However, his main emphasis was the service provision as opposed to profit. Munsterberg focussed on the psychological conditions of the work environment, in terms of achieving greater output and co-operation with management. Emerson published *The Twelve Principles of Efficiency* in 1913. His main argument stated ways of achievement as it was ideas as opposed to land, capital and labour that produced wealth. This is very much a notion that is coming to fruition in the twenty-first century with a drive towards the knowledge based society. He stated that it was ideas that should be rewarded, not the product. These combinations of thought process attached to the workplace culminated in an emphasis on the employee in their own personal achievement. Workplace health for the individual was communicated through self fulfilment in work. Exercising creativity and the ability to grow and develop is regarded as positive to the health of people at work.

Henry Fayol (1918) began with the observation that all forms of management in his native France, appear to have common features. They were made up of elements of planning, organising, commanding, co-ordinating and controlling. Fayol also set out a typology of organisations based on their primary functions:

- technical – production, manufacture, adaptation
- commercial – buying, selling, exchange
- financial – search for optimum uses of capital
- security – protection of property and persons
- accounting – stocktaking, balancing, costs, statistics
- managerial – planning, etc.

Each organisation type was then examined and analysed on the basis of the five elements of management to provide a detailed picture of the functions of each organisation, thus providing a blueprint for developing company guidelines – manuals of activity. He published *General and Industrial Management* in 1918. The work process and the division of labour was communicated in these specific elements.

Taylorism faced a great deal of opposition in its native America although much of Taylor's work was implemented in many enterprises around the world. However, the Western Electric Company in Chicago, were able to carry forward many of Taylor's ideas which eventually founded the Human Relations school.

Mayo, Roethlisberger and Dickson

Although Taylorism advocated profit as the main motivator of the work-force, the human relations thinkers advanced the notion that social interaction at work was of far greater importance.

The majority of experiments were initially performed using the Taylorist framework between 1924 and 1932. They sought to discover objective relationships between inputs and outputs, by altering lighting, wages, rest breaks and so forth. The intention was to produce measurable and directly related alterations in outputs. The researchers found no systematic relationships. It did not seem to matter what input or how input was altered, the output almost invariably rose. As a consequence, four main conclusions were drawn:

1   the work groups involved in the experiments were responding not to variations in conditions, but to the very fact of being treated as an experimental group with consequentially high status. They were acting in the ways they assumed they were supposed to react. In other words, the Hawthorne Effect was apparent;
2   the experience of working in a closely knit social group was in itself, a direct boost to productivity;
3   supervisors could play a crucial role in mediating between the demands of the company and the desires of the worker group;
4   the productivity increases provided repeated evidence of the 'latent energy' which work groups normally withheld through what the research team called their 'non-logical sentiments'. This however, could only be released through the right kind of management who operated along what they regarded as the more rational *logistics of cost and efficiency*. It was Mayo who interpreted this as the call of the isolated individual to be bound into the collective. Conformity to elite inspired norms was the normal path for the mass of subordinates in organisations who would only become anxious if left to decide for themselves.

Criticisms

Seivers (1984) argued that the social aspects of work only became important because Taylorism systematically shredded jobs of all inherent interest in pursuit of productivity gains. Gillespie (1991) extends this criticism in the sense that:

1 it continues to espouse a romantic notion of work, i.e. at some indeterminate time, all jobs had some intrinsic interest;
2 it focuses attention wholly on the job whereas the situation in which the job is executed is also important in defining the nature of the interest;
3 activities do not have intrinsic interest in the sense that they can be objectively assessed in isolation from the person undertaking the job. Job interests defined as those which the worker derives through interaction should be considered in establishing forms of job interest.

Hendrik de Man (1885–1953)

De Man was an early Marxist follower and Belgian socialist. He later abandoned Marxism for his own brand of socialism. Active in socialist movements in Belgium and Germany, de Man studied at the University of Leipzig and became Chair of Social Psychology at the University of Frankfurt in 1929. He wrote works on the psychology of socialism and on methods of Taylorism before his major work *Joy in Work* (1929) was translated by Eden Paul and Cedar Paul.

Joy in Work is based on de Man's experience in the socialist and trade union movements and his first hand observations of modern industrialism in Belgium, France, Germany, Russia, England and the United States. There are few investigators of the notion of work who have been involved with the working class and its movements, as well as in the academic world. De Man was unique in this respect.

Joy in Work is ostensibly a sociological study of work among German workers in the late 1920s based on a collection of 78 autobiographical reports on waged workers. This included blue collar and white collar occupations, skilled and unskilled workers, and a disproportionate number of workers in the trade union movement, and in the printing and metal working branches of industry. His specific findings are not nearly as significant as are his conceptual, analytical and philosophical discussions which flowed from his study. These discussions and insight into the social and psychological viewpoints of workers are still valid today, as they are based upon his perspective and knowledge of industrial society and its methods of work. Thus his book *Joy in Work* ranks as one of the major social/philosophical studies of the nature of work in modern industrial society.

The nature of work

De Man's study deals with questions about career, education, and changes of work. They include scope for initiative, variety in work, methods of payment, hygiene and safety, wages, vacations, work hierarchy, social and other aspects of the work environment. They deal with some of the positive and negative factors, and are very much a precursor of some of the work undertaken by Gardell (see Chapter 6), which enhance or hinder the joy in work. He also probed feelings about machines and tools, colleagues, superiors, the job in general and preferred leisure activities. The study dealt with the perceived connection between joy in work and participation in the works councils or in the trade unions, and whether membership in unions enhanced the joy in work. Finally, respondents were encouraged to specify how they thought their joy in work could be developed and increased. This included issues relating to changing the work process, the organisation of the firm, or the social order as a whole. The value of de Man's work is that it presents a conceptual framework for analysing the nature of work.

The premise taken by de Man emphasises that it is a mistake to look for forces favouring or hindering joy in work as concrete and measurable entities. The environment, equipment and the extant social order may all, in various combinations, allow the tendency toward satisfaction in work to have free scope or to be frustrated. He forcibly elucidates that it is the lived experience of the individual's participation in the work environment and work process which provides an insight into joy in work.

Influences of work on states of mind

In *Joy in Work*, de Man identifies a series of instincts which denote the experiences, whether positive or negative, that emanate in individuals during the work process.

- *Instinct of activity* – he states that inactivity is torment to a healthy individual. The normal form of activity is play in the child and work in the adult. The instinct of activity is directed toward the realisation of something which is mentally conceived. Thus when we observe issues of boredom and deskilling in the workplace, the impact on health of the individual and subsequent actions taken form an interesting link to stress (as in the work of Karasek, Theorell, and Marmot).
- *Instinct of play* – activity which has no other aim than the gratification of the doer is play. The instinct of play is to exert one's will which intensifies one's self esteem. We pass from play to work when value or utility is the motive of our action. We can feel the same joy in work that we do in play when we can give vent to a form of self expression and realise a subjective aim. Rhythm is the link connecting elements in work, play and art. Rhythm combats fatigue that arises out of repetitive work. Rhythm gives expression to a positive need and induces a pleasure which exists in play, where there is a gentle tension and relaxation and alteration of stimulation and repose. Control and the ability to plan and organise work contributes to the well being of the workforce.
- *The constructive instinct* – this is made up of three elements of creative

craftsmanship, orderly management and mechanical construction. The primary historical form of the constructive instinct was embodied in the craftsman of the Middle Ages. For the craftsman, plan and performance are one, beginning with a plan executed and modified as it is carried out by brain and hand. The tool is a prolongation of the hand and the hand is an appendage to the brain. The individual will find expression in work and every craft work is a work of art. The constructive instinct which aims at organisation and management in the industrial world is carried out by bureaucrats. In the craft world, it is carried out by craftsmen and women. In what is perceived to be ordinary circumstances, management is carried out rationally with rules and regulations. Organisation becomes a fetish regardless of its utility or results. In mechanical construction, joy in work for the worker depends upon the purposive functioning of this instrument of labour in the hands of the worker and there will be no joy in work if the worker is appendage to the machine. The same principle can be applied to computer technology in late twentieth century, be it the personal computer or cash register in the supermarket. The three varieties of the constructive instinct could be commingled, as with an electrical engineer who requires considerable intelligence for managing and organising the right to use machinery and maintaining the quality of the product.

- *Instinct of curiosity* – workers can find joy in work when they are gaining knowledge from their jobs. Working with machines can provide opportunities for inventing new methods of organisation and work management. Learning on the job or being transferred to learn other jobs can make work both satisfying and fulfilling.
- *Instinct of self assertion* – workers like to boast about their skills, physical strength or responsibility they have on their jobs. It is also the case that modern workers have instinct for asserting work reform and an improvement in the quality of working life (Levitan and Johnson 1982).
- *Possessive instinct* – many working people talk possessively of 'my machine' and if it performs well, they like it. If not, they hate it. Tools and machines are often given nicknames, peculiar to a particular trade or occupation.
- *Herd instinct* – this is the desire for social relationships on the job. For many workers, this aspect of the work environment can be one of the most important aspects of work which leads to job satisfaction. The chance to work in a large assemblage of persons in one workplace can be one of the conditions required for the gratification of the human need. This promotes a sense of well being and intensifies joy in work.

De Man provides a position on the need for subordination, aesthetic gratification and the consideration of self interest. He also writes of issues relating to the process of deskilling, along similar lines to the technological determinism hypothesis espoused by Marx and subsequent followers. He very much takes the line that later writers such as Frankenhauser and Gardell in that he states:

> ... people seek satisfaction as consumers – consumers not only of the material aspects of life, but also for the spiritual aspects of life, such as books, reading, culture, religion, community participation ... Generally seeking to improve their quality of life. As they improve their quality of life on the job, where they spend so much time, they want satisfaction in work through improvements in the way work is organised. They want improvements in the workplace which would promote initiative, more diversified types of work, more chances for constructive learning, more humanization, more interaction with others, greater democratization, participation in the way work is managed, and more chances to achieve self esteem on the job.
>
> de Man 1929, pp. 130–134

Neo-human relations school

The neo-human relations school began to develop after the Second World War at about the same time as ideas on socio-technical systems in the workplace. This school of thought became established through rejecting what they saw as simplistic models of human social behaviour. The main emphasis was on the achievement of *self actualisation* for the individual. That is, observations on how individuals realise their potential through the management of the organisation.

Maslow (1943) was one of the first to develop the idea of individual fulfilment through motivation at work. His ideas were based on a hierarchy of needs. To describe the condition of people at their best, Maslow chose Kurt Goldstein's term of self actualisation. For Goldstein, self actualisation, described any gratification or self fulfilment, whether it be the acquisition of food for hunger or knowledge for improvement. Maslow used the notion to describe the fact that self actualisation is rarely achieved until other complex needs lower down the hierarchy of personal requirements are fulfilled.

They are:

5 self actualisation
4 esteem, e.g. need for feeling personal worth; recognition, respect, admiration
3 belonging and love, e.g. feeling part of a group; able to give and receive love
2 safety, e.g. freedom from injury and illness
1 physiological, e.g. warmth, food, shelter

Self actualisation is the process whereby one realises the real self and works toward the expression of the self by becoming what one is capable of becoming. In other words, self actualisation is the process of making real the person's perception of the 'self'. It is a growth need. This implies that the person who has reached this summit has already taken care of the deficit needs and is in that state of psychological health where they begin the process of self realisation or becoming what they are capable of becoming. Not only is the mature individual driven to become what they can become, there is an inner compulsion to integrate interests, talents, and abilities to the point that the individual works toward becoming what they must become. The determinants here are the individual's own peculiar set of potentialities and the internally defined goals set by the individual.

For Maslow, the self actualised person is freed from the externally imposed deficit needs, and is ready to explore untried possibilities of the true self. The person type is characterised as spontaneous, creative and capable of achieving immense satisfaction from doing the thing that represents the realisation of their capabilities.

Maslow's basic premise is translated into issues concerning the individual and the organisational behaviour. Particular modes of operation within organisations can motivate or hinder the drive towards self actualisation. The impact on individuals is displaying either satisfaction or frustration in work. This is argued in the work of McGregor.

McGregor (1987) argued that the style of management adopted is a function of the manager's attitudes towards human nature and behaviour at work. He put forward two suppositions called Theory X and Theory Y which are based on popular assumptions about work, people and their behaviour at work. He argued that firms traditionally exhibited particular characteristics that:

1   most people had an inherent dislike of work;
2   coercion was therefore seen as necessary for compliance to work; and
3   most people preferred to be controlled rather than have autonomy.

This became Theory X. McGregor's theory was that this theory neglected the dynamic nature of human needs. As economic rewards satisfied material needs, so other, higher needs were ignited and subsequently higher forms of motivation are necessary. As a consequence, motivation becomes increasingly difficult because Theory X firms have no provision for coping with the new, higher needs of contemporary workers. McGregor argues, paradoxically, that the very success of capitalist management in the provision of wages, in itself, was of little motivational value. However, this is to assume that at a given level, material demands cease to increase and that universal human needs exist rather than needs which are socially and culturally constructed, hence transient.

This situation can be likened to Argyris' (1957) notions of the child/adult responsibilities, where individual development is premised upon the gradual accretion of responsibilities, organisations will thus only provide very limited roles for individuals, like the child, regardless of their abilities. The result is childish behaviour by adult employees frustrated at their treatment by the employers.

Theory Y provides a solution to the behavioural and motivational problems. The earlier assumptions of Theory X are reversed in that perhaps:

1   work is not disliked by everyone
2   coercion is not the only motivator
3   it is possible to provide organisational goals that fulfil the highest motivator, namely, self actualisation
4   responsible behaviour is a result of trust and avoidance of responsibility is a reaction to experiences that deny responsibility
5   creativity is widely dispersed throughout the population, even if few jobs require it

McGregor concludes that management's task is to develop *integrating* organisational procedures through which individuals can realise themselves through achieving organisational goals, that is, the goals as specified by management.

Criticisms

1   The ideas appear to be over-simplistic and do not account for the complexities of organisations in terms of group behaviour at different levels within the organisation. Coercion to conform may not always come through the management route. However, managerial ineptitude or laissez-faire can legitimise and thus validate some of the problems within the organisation. Harassment and bullying within the workplace has been identified as a feature of such behaviours (Adams 1992). It contains the situation and gives the group more power. One is left asking whose interest does this serve? (See arguments relating to organisational culture).
2   Repeats largely the issue that the reduction of responsibility can lead to alienation as initially demonstrated in the writings of Marx, Navarro and others.
3   Self actualisation is too easy a statement to make or to achieve within bureaucracies. The issues of job satisfaction, motivation, organisational culture, leadership and leader behaviour within the context of gender and race, needs to be fully explored.

Hertzberg's (1966) ideas on motivation were developed along similar lines to McGregor. However, he extended his interest to job satisfaction.

From his studies of over 200 engineers and accountants in nine different firms in Pittsburg, he concluded that there were hygiene and motivational factors which created dissatisfaction. Hygiene factors, denoted as the conditions, material rewards and security of work, are negative motivators in so far as their absence decreases productivity while their presence is merely the pre-condition for higher productivity. This has to be achieved through the positive motivation factors, which are symbolic and psychological rather than material, like status, advancement, and intrinsic job interest.

Systems theory focuses attention on the total work organisation. This approach was posited by von Bertalanffy (1951) who used the term to explain an organisation as consisting of systems that were interconnected and were mutually dependent on one another. This was derived from earlier ideas about society and the organic analogy. A malfunction in one part of the organisation would have an effect on other parts. This undoubtedly has an affect upon individuals within the organisation.

Socio-technical systems

This approach has also become linked with the idea of the development of social relations in the workplace, and draws on the work of Trist et al. (1951). Although largely a functionalist perspective, other ideas were developed from the original works of Trist and have subsequently been associated with other schools of sociological thought. For example, Walker (1952) and Guest's (1956) work describes the effects of the assembly line production method on employee behaviour. Woodward (1980) discusses the relationship between application of principles of organisation and business success. Sayles (1958) assesses the relationship between technology and the nature of work groups, and finally Blauner (1964) describes alienation in relation to different work technologies.

Contingency perspective

This theoretical approach was the next stage in evolution of organisational theory during the 1960s. Its origins lie in the work of Burns and Stalker (1961), Larwence and Lorsch (1967), and the Aston Studies (Pugh and Hikson 1976). It attempted to reduce the infinity of information implied in the systems approach down to a manageable level by focussing upon a delimited number of specific management problems, such as management structure, the issue of leadership, organisational bottlenecks, and so forth. Such problems, and their appropriate solutions, were regarded as contingent upon a small number of variables. Contrary to Taylor's assumption, there was no single best solution to resolve organisational problems but then neither did management have the freedom to do whatever it liked. Woodward (1958), for example, argued that although some degree of contingency existed, in so far as managers could choose between different forms of organisational structure, only those who chose the most appropriate structure, as determined by the technology of production, were likely to be successful. Thus contingency does not really relate to unrestricted choice nor to the level of uncertainty. In fact, the argument is one which attempts to remove contingency by specifying the conditions under which the success of particular organisations can be determined.

Contingency theory appeared to eliminate organisations of their occupants perspective and researchers began to explore the value of a perspective that attempted to resolve the subjective and active elements of organisations. *Action theory* appeared as a part of this development.

Silverman's (1970) pursuit of an action theory was drawn from the combined works of Weber, Shutz and Berger. Silverman argued that the action approach was a means of analysing social relations within organisations. Through social interaction, people could modify and possibly even transform social meanings which those involved assigned to their actions.

For example, whether failure to obey a superordinate's command was a manifestation of worker militancy, misunderstanding or just the beginnings of deafness depended not so much on what bosses or researchers saw happen but what the worker involved meant by his or her action. Occasionally, misunderstanding of the meaning of action was also possible so that the ultimate result of the interaction may not have been willed by any of the participants. Roy's (1973) ethnographic approach to work is seen as being able to demonstrate this process. Bowey (1976) has also suggested that the role, relationship, structure and process components of behaviour within organisations can be observed as part of the action approach.

Criticism

Action theories tended to be rather subjective and ignored the structural aspects of inequalities of power in work organisations.

Contemporary theories

Political organisation theories developed from two strands. The first is Child's (1972) *Strategic Choice* model which examines elite coalitions of managers who took positive action to ensure their interests prevailed over all others. The second, Lee and Lawrence (1985) draws upon the essentially political nature of organisational life, its innate contingency and the value of various strategies of influence to go well beyond the work of Child. Unfortunately, little room remains for analysis of the relationships between these human actors and the material and technological systems with which they interact. Power networks therefore, become restricted to social networks, rather than networks of human and non-human actors.

Salman (1986) also argues that values within organisations are inter-twined with the wider political environment. Therefore, any developments, either positive or negative within the organisation should be considered in relation to the political climate. He emphasised the need to go beyond Marx-ist explanations that reduce causes to the structural requirements of capit-alism and look at the complexities of organisational life.

Criticisms

The relationship between worker and employer is political, is about power, can mean deferred gratification, encourages subordination, stifles creativity and freedom of thought; reinforces powerless/powerful scenario.

The next stage in the evolution of organisation theory relates to the culture of organisations.

Organisational culture

Although popularised during the 1980s, studies of organisational culture entered the academic consciousness during the 1930s. The Hawthorne experiments undertaken in the Western Electric Company, Chicago, provides the earliest indication of the developments in organisational culture (Trice and Beyer 1993).

The Hawthorne experiments were particularly attentive to the relation-ships between productivity and the physical work environment. The initial experiments did not yield the results expected in pure technical terms and so behavioural scientists were employed to incorporate the initial results into a programme of ongoing research. This was initially spearheaded by Elton Mayo page 87 and his assistant W. Lloyd Warner who used anthropological methods to uncover the culture within Western Electric. This was the first occasion on which such methods were utilised within industry and led to the Bank Wiring Room Observation Study in 1931–1932. The main purpose of the study was to determine how work group cultures affected worker beha-viour and productivity in a specific work setting.

Warner began a new phase in the cultural studies of organisations.

Observations and interviews were aimed at describing three kinds of social relations occurring in the room: the technical, the social and the ideological ... technical relations arranged the flow of materials to machines, tools and their input. The social structure organised the work, both formally in terms of specific designated relations, and informally in terms of those friendships and cliques that naturally formed outside the formal, prescribed relationships. The third kind of relations, the ideological, concerned the workers' culture – their shared beliefs and understandings regarding the work setting.

Trice and Beyer 1993, p. 24

Although much of the literature credits Mayo and Warner with the development of studies in organisational culture, other authors imply that it was Roethlisberger and Dickson who analysed the data and undertook a full account of the research studies (Trahair 1984).

Gardner popularised the study of industrial anthropology at the University of Chicago Business School during the 1940s and wrote the first textbook which took account of the cultural perspectives of work organisations, *Human Relations in Industry* (Gardener 1945). Whyte (1948) brought another perspective to the study of organisational culture and symbolism. Its primary focus related to the informal social structure of organisations.

During the 1950s and 1960s in the US and UK, much of the efforts of the studies of organisations generally focussed on quantitative studies. As for the study of culture, it moved on with reference to the wider society, led primarily by Levi-Strauss. However, there were a few studies of note that persisted in organisational culture.

Selznick (1949) described the interactions of affected communities and the fledgling Tennessee Valley Authority in terms of how institutions respond to changing circumstances. He used the term institution to describe the notion that organisations were more than the sum of technical operations. The Tavistock Institute (in England) began to do research on organisations as cultural systems, also during this period. They attempted to introduce values about employee participation in the decision making process (an idea taken up by the Karolinska Institute, Sweden by Gardell et al. in the 1960s and 1970s). Also, Caudhill (1958) studied the day-to-day personal relations of doctors, ward personnel, and patients in a psychiatric hospital.

Dalton's (1959) studies rested on subcultures which emerge from workers needs and how they operated informally to govern the operations within companies. He uncovered the dynamics of the social life of organisations which emerged amongst the formal rules and regulations. The most determined and sustained efforts were made by Roy (1952, 1953, 1954, 1960) who used participant observation to study culture within small work groups and yielded results that were similar to those of the Hawthorne studies.

Henry (1963), made his contribution by studying the public school as a transmitter of cultural values such as thrift, competitiveness, cleanliness and industry. It was during the late 1960s that a breakthrough came from cultural researchers, which had been largely neglected in organisation and management studies. In the US, a team of researchers led by Trice published their observations of personnel practices, interpreting them as cultural rites and ceremonials (Trice et al. 1969). Later, Mintzberg (1973, 1975) popularised the use of qualitative techniques for studying organisations through the managerial lens. In the UK, Turner's (1971) contribution of the period was an exploration of the substance and forms of organisational cultures. However, it was Pettigrew (1973), who recovered the impetus of the study of organisational culture with ICI, using qualitative methods of data collection.

So far this has been a historical trip through the main developments in the study of organisational culture. For the most part, up to the late 1970s the recognition of specific studies were grouped with a rationalist framework.

In 1977 two articles were published that criticised rationalist approaches to organisations. Meyer and Rowan's *Institutionalised Organisations: Formal Structure as Myth and Ceremony* treated rationalised and organisational principles as symbols of modernity and efficiency. In addition to this, Lynne Zucker's *The Role of Institutionalisation in Cultural Persistence*, explored the microprocesses surrounding the construction of modern, rationalised organisational practices. These new theoretical developments turned the rationalist approach to organisations on its head by arguing that supposedly universal precepts are merely abstractions from social practices that emerged for complex historical reasons. It was underlined that the study and understanding of social processes as they arise within the organisation was the way forward. Between March 1983 and October 1984, five major conferences on corporate culture and folklore and symbolism were held. These conferences stimulated a renewal of confidence in the study of organisations, particularly culture.

Organisational ideologies

Harrison (1972) was the first to develop a basic taxonomy of organisational cultures. They were later popularised by Handy (1985) and comprised the following: power, role, task and person. It is noted that few organisations are one or other type of culture, they usually exhibit characteristics of each. Handy's categorisation of types of culture have been found to be beneficial because:

1　it presents a number of different cultures within organisations
2　it highlights the difficulty of defining cultures in a clear way
3　it provides profound implications of the cultural approach to organisations

These implications have been identified by other authors.

Deal and Kennedy (1983) argued that behaviour, is shaped by shared values, beliefs and assumptions about the way an organisation should operate, how rewards should be distributed, the conduct of meetings, even how people should dress. They do not consider behaviour within organisations is a result of reaction to intrinsic and extrinsic motivators. Also, the culture-excellence school observe that there are specific cultures which relate to organisational success.

Sathe (1983) argued that culture guides the actions of an organisation's members without the need for detailed instructions or long meetings to discuss how to approach particular issues or problems; it also reduces the level of ambiguity and misunderstanding between functions and departments. In effect, culture shapes the purpose and context of the organisation.

Barratt concludes that 'values, beliefs and attitudes are learnt, can be managed and changed, and are potentially manipulative by management' (1990, p. 23). Thus as Schein (1985) observes, managers have an important influence on the organisation's cultural make-up. However, one criticism of Handy's categorisation of culture, is that he fails to give sufficient weight to the influence of natural cultures which predominate in individual countries (Hofstede 1991).

What is organisational culture?

There have been a number of ideas put forward about the organisation, its operation and its people. However, an organisation's significance and real purpose (beside the obvious notion of the provision of goods and services), needs further exploration.

Silverman (1970) contended that organisations are societies in miniature and can therefore be expected to show evidence of their own cultural characteristics. This may be the case, but, it implies that within these mini-societies there exists conflict, consensus, interactions that lead to behavioural change, and the *rules for living* are reflected within the organisation as in wider society.

Culture defines how those in the organisation should behave in a given set of circumstances. It affects all, from the most senior manager to the humblest clerk. In relation to the behavioural aspects, Turner (1971) observed that cultural systems contain elements of 'ought' which prescribe forms of behaviour or allow behaviour to be judged acceptable or not.

Organisational culture ... [is a] ... system of shared values, norms and routines that manifests itself through the rich tapestry of anecdote, mythical fairy-tale, all of which serve to communicate and reinforce shared values and beliefs within an organisation.

Peters and Waterman 1982

Schein's (1985) view extends this perception in that organisational culture is generally perceived as:

... a basic set of assumptions which a given group has invented, discerned or developed in learning to cope with its problem of external adaptation and internal integration, which have worked well enough to be considered valid, and therefore ... [are] ... taught to new members on the correct way to perceive, think and feel in relation to those problems. [These assumptions] ... lie behind the values ... and determine the behaviour patterns and visible artefacts such as architecture, office layout, dress codes and so on ....

Schein 1985, p. 14

Schein's ideas are formulated through his interest in anthropology and group dynamic theory. Leadership is also regarded as an important element in his thinking about organisational culture. He states that popular notions of culture merely reflect culture as opposed to providing a description of the essence of culture. He argues therefore that the culture of an organisation is embedded in its preconsciousness and beliefs about human nature. At another level, culture manifests as values which are testable only by social consensus. The values of an organisation relate to what works, and how things ought to be done. When a value is agreed upon by a group, the group begins the process of cognitive transformation, in which the value becomes a belief or assumption. These assumptions are taken for granted rather than debatable. The other aspect of this notion relates to what is on the surface. Schein calls these artefacts, i.e. technology, art, behavioural pattern, reports, documents outlining the achievements of an organisation, its written rules.

Elements of organisational culture

The fundamental elements of organisational culture are observed and monitored in many ways. Beckhard (1969) identified what it meant to have a healthy organisation. This extended to positive correlations found between culture and organisational effectiveness (Ouchi 1981; Deal and Kennedy 1982; Denison 1984). Information sharing, delegation, results oriented, developmental, egalitarian, employee-centred cultures are believed to enhance adaptiveness, productivity, innovation and performance (Kanter 1983; Denison 1984; Walton 1985).

The strength of cultures within organisations are also seen as important. Wilkins and Ouchi (1983) suggested that strong cultures (clan mechanisms) may enhance organisational efficiency only under conditions of uncertainty and ambiguity (hence high 'transactions' costs), stability of membership, and reasonably equitable and inescapable reward systems. If these conditions do not exist, markets or hierarchies may better meet the firm's need for internal integration.

Organisational cultures can cushion and reinforce behaviours in the process of socialisation. These can be positive or negative, advertent or inadvertently impact upon the individual. One element of this feature is the rise and ceremonials within organisation, often displayed on the arrival of the newcomer or in an attempt to make the high achiever uncomfortable (Trice and Roman 1971). The familiar rites of passage and rites of degradation force particular responses from individuals (Garfinkel 1956; Fortes 1962; Trice and Beyer 1984; see also Chapter 1).

Post-modernist paradigms regard organisations as reactions against inherently destabilising forces (Cooper and Burrell 1988). Organisations are not progressive and evolutionary. The organisation threatens humanity with absolute control derived from spreading the tentacles of control over resources and ideas, as well as exercising its control through legitimisation in terms of rationality and progress. This is based on the premise that reason produces human progress.

The post-modernist view of organisations is generally one of dissensus, uncertainty and instability. This notion is developed by Derrida (1973, 1978) who states that organisations are developed not as mechanisms to advance human control but to mask the world of uncertainty. Derrida and others such as Foucault, deny the plausibility of any group being in control, for to be in control presumes a rational intent and means to effect such intent. In short, post-modernists start from the assumption that organisations are the results of reactive processes, attempts to delimit the disaggregating complexity and confusing reality of everyday existence.

The uncertainty and fragility of social life becomes a stimulus to construct reality-distancing mechanisms: organisations are facades constructed not to advance human control but to obscure the reality that we have no control.

In turn, this reproduction of the practices that sustain the precarious, but taken for granted, nature of the world ultimately prevents us from recognising the nature of the social world (Knights 1989).

Meaning is imputed by the observer on the organisation. For Derrida, meaning found within the organisation is an attempt to create reality (Cooper 1989).

Criticisms

1 Observing an organisation in purely linguistic terms avoids the reality of social relations and group processes within the workplace, unless of course language is placed within a context where actions of the performers are also taken into consideration.

2 Derrida implies that the rules and structures of an organisation are within the eye of the beholder. Apparent rather than real.

Foucault's ideas

Foucault's ideas on organisations may be interpreted through his views on society. He argues that contemporary society is maintained by surveillance on the body and through discipline which is built into the framework of the institutions of the society and hence, organisations. So like prisoners, workers must always be visible to their controllers and the minutiae of daily life is legitimately ordered and observed from above and written up, not into personal details, but into bureaucratic case notes. Subjectivity is systematically stripped by an organisation and a model of normality is reconstituted from the elements; anyone deviating from this model is the subject of further dissection by society's human scientists, the self appointed judges of *normality*.

Foucault's ideas are derived from the notion of networks of power. Power is a partially stable network of alliances amongst people within the workplace. People are constructed by power but do not have power. Power then is not the property of any individual or group, still less can it be discovered within structures. Power then, should be configured as a relation between subjects, the microphysics of everyday life. It is 'capillary power' and is exercised within the social body rather than above it (Foucault 1980, p. 39). He underlines that not all subjects are equal with the network of power relations which defines them. The resources of power are unequally distributed and this inequality is frequently buttressed by the strategies employed by resource rich subjects. Thus people with power are those with particular resources that the organisation can draw upon for its own purpose, whether they be a particular range of skills or social contacts or access to physical resources.

For Foucault, those who resist the constraints of the power network, are disciplined, the greater the resistance, the more discipline is bestowed upon the individual (Burrell 1988). Control imposed upon the individuals is maintained. This may take the form of the power network or through electronic forms such as computer technology.

Criticisms

1   Organisations within the Foucauldian framework emphasise inclusion and exclusion of subjects within society.
2   Organisations reinforce subordination of individuals. As there is no hierarchy in the power network it may impinge upon those in any sector of the organisation.
3   Values, beliefs and attitudes are extremely subjective and can be a handicap for progress within the organisation in terms of productivity and progress. The power network will exercise its force in order to maintain the status quo.

The changing nature of work

The last 20 years of the twentieth century was characterised by some as post-Fordism. The notion of post-Fordism can be described as '... the progressive decentralisation of production under conditions of rising flexibility and centralised strategic control'. (Hoggett 1990).

Post-Fordist tendencies have been observed in multi-skilling and team working in Japanese factories, and the growth of lean production (Womack et al. 1990). It has also been seen as job enrichment through upskilling and increasing autonomy in the German automobile production systems (Lane 1989) and in the artisanal production of the 'Third Italy' (Poire and Sabel 1984). Others, who's views may be more in keeping with Aglietta, see a hybrid between mass productivity and flexible specialisation, the emphasis being the new ways of working which are still in process of development (Hirst and Zeitlin 1990).

In the UK, the notion of post-Fordism may be interpreted in three distinct ways. Firstly, the erosion of national pay bargaining structures so creating a more flexible labour market in terms of hours of work and pay. Secondly, the promotion of externalisation meaning external decentralisation, perhaps with the exception of local management of schools, and thirdly, the weakening of local government and service structures into a fragmented series of units, as in the NHS where we saw during the 1990s the development of trusts, fund holding and non-fund holding establishments. The aim being to initiate greater competition between service providers and at the same time encourage greater efficiency, effectiveness and improvements in service quality (Atkinson and Meager 1986).

The notion of post-Fordism, however, is derived from a number of schools of thought. The approach known as *regulation*, is advocated by Aglietta (Jessop 1990). The focus of his work rests on an analysis of the ways in which capitalism at an international level continues to thrive and survive. The process involves the dynamics of accumulation and the mode of regulation to prevent crises occurring between mass production and capitalism. New forms of working were developed to preserve capital at the cost of labour. In other words, more flexible working patterns, new forms of managerialism and reduction in the negotiating powers of trades unions had become a feature of the organisation of work – which Aglietta calls neo-Fordism (Jessop 1991).

The second approach, from the *institutionist* school, focuses on the way markets become fragmented. Technological change is central to the alterations in work and working relationships (Clutterbuck 1980). Atkinson and Meager (1986) also see technology as the main cause of increasing flexibility. The flexible firm heralded the advent of core and peripheral workers within organisations where there is a clear divide between permanent, highly skilled and well paid staff and those who are on short term contracts, work part time and are more readily dispensable.

The approaches offered by the institutionist and regulatory schools are closed, technological determinist perspectives which limit the development of analysis to technology, equals crises, equals a more streamlined workforce, equals misery for those on the periphery. The onion peel effect. Whereas Aglietta offers an explanation which is partial and provides room for exploration of the power relations in work, and at the same time the political versus economic dimensions and how they impinge upon work on a macro level. In other words, the dynamics are in a process of evolution (Hyman 1988; Sayer 1989).

Criticisms

Ideas relating to post-Fordism have been criticised on empirical and theoretical grounds. Firstly, the issue of a divide between mass production and specialisation is seen as too simplistic. There is evidence to state that the two can co-exist under capitalism (Taplin 1989; Wood 1993). It is also not entirely clear that Fordism was ever a pervasive generic production system as is claimed, as some durable and non-durable goods manufacture involves small batch production. Also, sufficient evidence exists to demonstrate that what flexible specialisation often entails is a more sophisticated use of labour that masks intensification of effort, thus making it indistinguishable from neo-Fordism. Even in regions where its successes have been proclaimed, such as Italy and Japan, intensification of effort rather than job enrichment are often the norm for production workers (Lovering 1990; Taplin 1995).

Another criticism rests on the demand driven technological innovation, i.e. market saturation and subsequent segmentation, places too much emphasis on influential approaches without questioning why alternative responses might have occurred. For Poire, Sabel and Atkinson, changing technology over determines the process of production and hence alterations in the labour market.

What is considered to be the post-Fordist ways of working, compound, rather than eliminate, inequalities. Any restructuring would seem to consist mainly of the reduced impact of institutionalised compromises between employers and their workforces as collectives. Labour is increasingly regulated instead through markets, in the form of set socially differentiated labour markets. Ideologies of gender, race and age are deeply embedded in this structure. The changes made for economic reasons impinge upon categorising a labour market into qualified/unqualified, skilled/unskilled. Social categories such as gender, race and class are major axes of differences here since they are closely associated with access to educational qualifications and enabling or constraining circumstances as outside the workplace.

Given that many companies have survived by acquiring rather than training labour, existing social divisions in the labour market have been exploited rather than challenged. Men still monopolise the scarce and best paid occupations, women fill the jobs where they have less bargaining power, many black women fill those where they have least (Lovering 1990).

The European Commission (Bosch 1995) presents a slightly broader concept of flexibilisation. It involves the notions of promotion and participation. Legal standards alone are not able to support flexibility. They see the need for stability of employment which also means an investment in training. Decentralised decision making is to be extended as an expression of a new division of labour between levels of work regulation. Socially acceptable and respectable arrangements are to be encouraged for employees. Flexibility is seen as an attempt to reintegrate work tasks and in the introduction of teamwork.

When applied to the welfare state, Jessop (1991) has underlined what he considers to be the elements of post-Fordism. They are:

1 flexibilisation in welfare services
2 a new balance between public and private sectors
3 the reduction in the cost of welfare. These are tailored to the needs and preferences of the consumer, flattened management structures, labour process and employment patterns and increased regulation of welfare services, as well as a significant shift away from state funded provision

Although Jessop's views have been severely criticised he can be seen to have had a vision. Firstly, there are examples within the British health service where flexibilisation has occurred. Leicester Royal Infirmary, faced with budgetary difficulties and increasing demands on the service from patients and treatment costs, in 1993 changed its way of working. There was large investment in the training and development of staff, it introduced the process of re-engineering in primary health care and altered its operating theatres and ENT services in terms of team working and flexible working patterns for staff. A patient's council was also introduced to provide feedback on developments for their members. Staff morale was improved and jobs protected. Efficiency in terms of care and treatment has expanded by 50%. Similar work was undertaken in Denmark and Germany (European Commission 1998).

Under the 1990 reforms with the introduction of the internal market, the NHS and the private sector were also competing for the same market with the rise of cheaper and more readily available healthcare insurance schemes. Health promotion services were also left with positions of becoming integrated with commissioning authorities, being trust providers or self-funded/ managed independent units. The dispersal has subsequently increased into primary care groups in the last part of the century.

It will be interesting to see the developments in time in terms of power structures within those organisations or whether there is a return to more functionalist notions of interdependency within organisations.

New forms of work organisation

New forms of work organisation is a concept and philosophy of the market. It is a late twentieth century phenomenon used by companies to implement a host of strategic decisions that are taken in response to new challenges and pressures of globalisation. It is characterised by the notions of efficiency and effectiveness within the workplace. Indeed, the main message that appears to be communicated includes:

1 improving innovative capacity
2 improving operative efficiency
3 improving customer responsiveness and levels of customer service
4 adopting a quality management strategy
5 maximising benefits from investment in new technologies
6 re-engineering service delivery in public sector organisations

It is intended to be people centred in relation to issues of participation within the decision making processes of organisations. Whether this is the actuality in terms of real benefits, promoting well being and reducing alienation is as yet largely untested.

The internal processes of the organisation and forms of working enable, on the surface, the developments that a century of researchers have stated as a real need within the workplace. Companies participating in pilot schemes to develop or enhance the new forms of working such as Fasson, Scandinavian PC Systems, Brabantia and Leicester Royal Infirmary have attempted reduction in management layers, flexible working hours, and semi-autonomous work schemes (European Commission 1998). However, greater working between trades unions and management will be required to create a working environment where the needs of the individual and the needs of the market are balanced.

New forms of work also include home working and self employment. Today, approximately 14 million men and 11.5 million women make up the total workforce in Britain, this includes the self employed, trainees and the armed forces. The Labour Force Survey (LFS 1996) showed that 3.2 million people were self employed, 242,000 on training programmes and approximately 2.3 million unemployed.

The advent of self employment has seen an increase in almost a decade from 7.3 per cent to 12.7 per cent and there has been a decrease in full time employment of men from 58.1 per cent to 50.5 per cent. There has been no substantial alteration in the number of women in full time employment at 24 per cent. There has, however, been an increase in part time working for both men (from less than 1 per cent to 4.6 per cent) and women from 17.1 per cent to 20.3 per cent.

The issue of working hours however, is much the same as the 1960s. The average number of hours worked per week is 33.2 hours. Respondents who described themselves as full time self employed worked more hours per week than the average, being 42.4 hours rather than full time employees who work 36.7 hours. The situation is reversed for part time workers who work more hours per week on average than the self employed (15 and 11.8 hours respectively.) The UK is unique in having a very wide distribution of working hours, with almost 16 per cent working more than 48 hours a week. This is just over twice the average for the European Union.

There are now in Britain, some 2.7 per cent of people working from their own homes. The majority are concentrated in what may be considered to be the service sector. Almost 75 per cent are in managerial, professional, technical, clerical or secretarial occupations. Approximately 50 per cent of all home workers are self employed. The benefits or drawbacks to this form of working has yet to be assessed in terms of well being and health of the individual.

Chapter 5

Theoretical perspectives of workplace health improvement

In Chapter 2, we saw some of the major historical contributions to the evolution of workplace health. This was underlined specifically in terms of legislation, the public health movement and commentary of the conditions of work during the nineteenth and early twentieth century. The trade unions have also contributed with their mass of evidence from their fellow workers which eventually led to the development of the occupational health service in Britain.

In this chapter, some of the theoretical contributions to the movement in the latter part of the twentieth century are discussed. Specific themes and perspectives are explored in relation to health problems at work and approaches for health improvement.

The historico-political approach

The historico-political approach generated a series of ideas about workplace health (WPH) based on Marx's macro-political assumptions, namely class, economics and capitalism. The impact on the individual worker is marked out by components of this political process. Although the process of evolution falls short of expression about notions of gender and 'race', they provide a useful approach to understanding political process and action at work.

In the Marxist tradition, already established in Chapter 4, production is expressed as the organiser of society. The place that the individual has in the world of production determines their place in the world of consumption, exchange, distribution and legitimisation, as well as their health. Needless to say, what happens on other levels – ideological and political, has an autonomy of its own, and also has great importance in explaining health and medicine. These movements and levels influence production and are influenced by it, but they are created and articulated within a whole, a social formation or society, where production is a determinant movement that characterises the social formation. Much of the work from this perspective is undertaken by Navarro and Waitzkin.

Vincente Navarro

Navarro has written from a perspective that underlines the effect of capitalism and industrial development upon health. His approach is decidedly Marxian in essence and his preoccupation rests with the impact of capitalism on society at a macro level and at the same time, provides a theoretical perspective which intelligently provides an opinion on health and illness in the workplace. The work has focused specifically on the industrial process as a constraining force upon the worker and that the medical profession reinforces this strain by supporting management views on accidents and compensation issues. In *Work, Ideology and Science: The Case of Medicine* he takes a broad view of the connection between work and health. There is evidence to suggest that the connection between capital, labour and ill health emanate from within society (Navarro 1980). This contributed to the notion that conflict between capital and labour, and the problems which can occur as a result of increased productivity, places an imbalance on the demands of labour.

The worker is encapsulated in an oppressive system whereby the dominant ideology of the specific work process forces the worker to accept a system that places them at a disadvantage. Navarro claims the worker is unconscious of the specific regime when lured into the environment where there is a trade-off between profit margin and individual income.

Occupational medicine reinforces the dominant ideology in the workplace by holding its primary task in identifying for company owners, the size and nature of the damage which requires compensation. This is the damage which emanated from the process of industrialisation and 'selection' for work within the capitalist framework. Doctors were charged with the task of defending managerial interests and detracting from the damage created at the workplace.

> The struggle was and still continues to be between labour, which demanded a higher compensation, and capital, denying for as long as possible that there was any relationship between work, disease and death.
>
> Navarro 1980, p. 529

In his observation of injury statistics in the USA over a 30 year period between 1940 and 1970, Navarro claimed that there were substantial increases in each decade of the stated period. There was a clear relationship found between higher productivity and increased accidents in the workplace. Particularly notable during the intervening period was the increase in reported disease, stress and malaise in the workplace which had a great impact on the life of workers and their families (Navarro 1980). Workplaces are seen as sites of struggle in relation to economy, productivity and competition, where the worker is found at the centre of power relationships which often conflict with their health (see Chapter 1).

The effect that was brought about through constraining forces in the workplace is underlined in this quote which depicts a hierarchical division of labour.

> A primary characteristic of work is that it is controllers ... [Who] ... increasingly shape the nature of work to optimize their pattern of control over the productive process, in the individual producers, and the collectivity of producers ....
>
> Navarro 1980, p. 526

This particular process of control over the workforce is characterised by three primary functions. The first relates to *compartmentalisation*. This involves reducing work tasks into more narrow focus and direction. This can be seen as constraining for the worker who prefers to express some creativity in their work and would like to be presented with the opportunity to see the completed product. Compartmentalisation is restrictive and controlling for the individual worker.

The second is placing the workforce into positions which reinforce and reproduce the class relations in society, known as *hierarchilisation*. The hierarchy within an organisation, consisting of managers, supervisors, and shop floor workers, can be seen to be akin to broader society in terms of earning capacity, wages/salary, status and the extent of responsibility which relate on a basic level to the working, petty bourgeoise and middle classes. This particular level of focus related to the industrial factory system that predominated during the 1950s to 1970s across the western world. The issue of class, within the wider society was replicated in the work environment.

The third aspect of the process relates to *expropriation*. The term describes a situation where workers have much less influence and control over their work, its design, its process or any of the products they are intended to create. The effect is regarded as totalitarian and is commented on as:

> [A] ... set of authoritarian relations where class – the bourgeoisie – controls that process of production and work and the other – the working class – doesn't, is what Marx called dictatorship of the bourgeoisie, understanding as such not a specific political form of government but rather an overwhelming dominance and control which the bourgeoisie has over the means and process of production.
>
> Navarro 1980, pp. 526–527

The process mentioned was very much a feature of industrial organisation up to the late 1970s. It ran parallel with the drive towards increased efficiency and productivity of the worker. Indeed, it emphasises that employers and employment processes so functioned to extract as much from the worker as possible for little reward. The absence of alternative models of productivity underlined the problems experienced. Ill health arose from the monotonous impact of industrialisation and technologisation of the workplace which places workers at a disadvantage.

For Navarro, the expropriation of health that takes place at the workplace is further reproduced by the expropriation of health that occurs in the communities, in the environment, in the family, in all components of everyday life. The articulation of workplace related struggles with non-work related issues, and the articulation of forms of direct with indirect democracy, are key issues for the resolution of the exploitation and expropriation of health of the majority of people.

The fragmentation of the worker's tasks often reduces their responsibility, loosens their control and surveillance. The social position of the individual is altered and they become devalued. This is known as the proletarianisation of the workforce, i.e. reducing their skills, control over their work. '... this situation creates enormous dissatisfaction, as expressed in high turnover rates, absenteeism, resistance to the prescribed workplace, indifference, neglect and overt hostility to management ...'. (Navarro 1982, p. 16).

In the early 1990s a slightly different set of circumstances occurred with similar effect of proletarianisation. This actually affected those higher up the hierarchy of the organisation in management whose positions were being devalued with performance related pay, short term contracts and constant surveillance through charters and quality assurance initiatives (Thompson 1990; Thompson and Warhurst 1998), the structure of the organisation being altered.

Navarro makes several claims on the behaviour of the capitalist class:

> ... An important one is to make workers accept the situation as a 'given', the inevitable outcome of 'progress' or 'industrialization' or whatever. The social relations of work are considered as unavoidably determined by the technical requirements of the labour process.
>
> Navarro 1982, p. 16

Another part of the process of the devaluation of the worker, in the removal of control, is the isolation of the individual from other workers.

This isolation reaches its extreme form in home piecework, where individuals are contracted to work in their own homes. Management shifts whole processes of production from the factory to individual workers' homes as a way of debilitating labour and avoiding collective action by labour. The 'diffused' factory or place of work sometimes also referred to as the 'factory without walls', was indeed a type of capitalist intervention aimed at weakening and dividing the working class and isolating the workers. This was a predominant feature in blue collar industries in the US and British manufacturing up to the mid-1970s.

The introduction of the new technology in the late 1970s and early 1980s contributed to the rolling and psychologically corrosive notion of deskilling. According to Navarro, the introduction of new technologies had contributed to other hazards to health for the worker. New skills were invariably required in a new economic and technological regime. This can subsequently, lead to the process of deskilling. For example, the establishment and expansion of the producer services employed large numbers of new professional banking, insurance, and communications. This was a highly intensive labour process. The introduction of computers and microprocessors has seen a superspecialisation of the few at the detriment of the larger workforce. This similar process along with task specialisation has also been seen in the manufacturing industries.

Deskilling has led to stress, psychological problems in increased risk in cardiovascular disease (Gardell 1983; Marmot and Theorell 1988; see Chapter 1).

The economic system of capitalism is regarded as problematic for the worker in many ways: Firstly, it encourages the increasing intensity of the work for the individual worker. For example, forcing the worker to operate at a more rapid pace, introducing changes in the means of work, the organisation of work and specialisation of the workers the (*relative surplus value*). Secondly, these increases or alterations in the pace of change herald such problems as excessive fatigue and stress. Thirdly, the introduction of novel means of production, e.g. in terms of new machinery and other forms of technology, under developing workers through poor training, may lead to new exposures to risks from accidents and toxic materials. Indeed it can be stated that '... we can speak of absolute expropriation of health when the loss of health is due to the appropriation of absolute surplus value, the predominant form of exploitation in underdeveloped capitalist countries'. (Navarro 1982, p. 16).

In *The Labour Process and Health: a Historical Materialist Interpretation*, Navarro expounds a more developed view of the problems of work and health:

... the analysis of a social whole (composed of several movements – production, consumption and exchange – and several levels – economic, politico-judicial and ideological), taking production as the starting point in that analysis. In other words, the basis of any society is what is produced, how it is produced, and how it is distributed. All production is characterized by two inseparable elements: The Labour process, which is any process of transformation of a definitive object (either natural or already worked upon) into a definitive product, a transformation affected by a definite human activity, using definite instruments of labour, and the relations of production which are the concrete historical forms in which the labour process is realized.

Navarro 1982, pp. 8–9

In terms of developing a position of the effects of work upon the individual, he communicates a multilevel approach to analysis. A set of ideas which communicate activity within the macro political context of society is the point of departure when discussed alongside the labour process.

The means of labour in the most broadest sense are all the material conditions that do not interfere directly with the process of transformation (of an object) which are indispensable for its realisation. Without the 'means of labour' work cannot be done, there must be an environment in which 'work' takes place. Further credence to the means of labour is provided in Navarro's analysis:

The means of labour can be analyzed in terms of their technical sophistication or as an expression of specific social relations. From the first perspective, areas to look at include the physical effort needed to execute the work; the interaction between workers, the objects of work, and the means of labour; and the degree of control that the workers have over the means of work and over the process of work. Each of these different components of the labour process is an expression of the social relations that created it.

Navarro 1982, p. 11

Navarro very much adheres to the view that the means of labour are a part of the labour process which is two-fold, the initial relating to technicalities – the physical resources and effort in producing work. The second aspect lies in the interaction, the relations between and among the workforce '... the instruments of work, such as machines, dictate the rhythm of work and limit the decision making of the workers. Both increase under certain conditions, the accident proneness not of the worker, but the instrument of labour'. (Navarro 1982, p. 11).

These elements provide the very clues for the work process and in turn the impact they have upon the individual and the organisation. The issue of labour power was also of concern. Human energy and labour power for Navarro, relate to concepts which are radically different from the realised work, which is only the expression or expenditure of that labour power. By confusing the concepts, classical economy was not capable of realising the origin of capitalist exploitation, i.e. the creation of value. It presents the view that wages are the price of the work realised by the workers, very much the old Taylorist notion.

> There are two different modes of increasing the surplus value, which correspond to two different forms of appropriation of labour power. Each form, in turn, implies different forms of wearing out the worker and expropriating his health. One mode is by increasing the overall time of work. If a worker who produces in four hours, the value equivalent to the value of his labour power, works another four hours, he produces a surplus value of 100 per cent.
>
> Navarro 1982, p. 12

The implication here being that the lives of workers were shortened every time their hours of work increased.

Alienation and its impact on worker health

Navarro interpreted Marx's ideas on alienation directly by stating that alienation was a condition of separation of the worker from his labour power (see Chapter 4). Alienation is seen as the outcome of social relations that emerge from waged labour. The subsequent response within the individual worker can emerge in a number of situations:

> ... several studies have concluded that workers see work as a major determinant of life situation and self esteem, far more important than non-work abilities such as education and leisure pursuits. To have an interesting, rewarding job is reported in these studies as being one of life's most important goals. Work contributes substantially to the construction of one's personality. Unless these needs are satisfied at the workplace, the individual experiences a basic frustration that manifests itself in different efforts to achieve adjustment.
>
> Navarro 1982, p. 17

Although Navarro provides an interesting framework for analysis, it remains on the macro political level and therefore incomplete in terms of reaction and response within the individual. It does, however, form the basis upon which new developments were made in pushing the boundaries forward. Other researchers have taken these components – self esteem, notion of work and leisure, construction of personality and issues of frustration, and developed positions of their own (Gardell; Gustavsen; Syme; Johnson and Johansson).

Criticisms

1   The issue of class in these sets of circumstances requires more thought within the context of late twentieth century management structure. Middle management has experienced the same expropriation with flattened organisational structures. The situation has become one of the individual performance and worth in the organisation. Class is still relevant as one major component in the issue of expropriation, but the means of domination has altered.

2   Exploration of the concept of alienation requires extension. With the advent of new forms of work organisation, it can be argued that the forces of capitalism are an even greater inherent feature of workplaces, but the process of alienation emerges from additional sources of domination, not simply class position or relations. Group process and a thirst for greater material gain reinforces rather than challenges the situation that becomes one of alienation at work, as seen in the work of Adams (1992) and more recently the TUC where the impact on health can be detrimental. It appears that professionals, the professional classes, are too experiencing alienation in the workplace. So the predominant feature of late twentieth century workplaces in relation to this concept is that the boundaries have not been so much defined between classes, but rather removed in the clamour for survival.

Howard Waitzkin

Waitzkin draws upon historical works of Engels, Virchow and Allende to highlight the fact that the historical and political processes within society contribute to and reinforce the likelihood of illness at work.

Conditions in which people were forced to live and work in, invariably caused sickness and early death during the nineteenth century. Environmental pollution, airborne infection, infant mortality and overcrowding in industrial cities made for a potent reminder of the living conditions in industrial cities.

> The individual in society is not an abstract entity; one is born, develops, lives, works, reproduces, falls ill, and dies in strict subjection to the surrounding environment, whose different modalities create diverse modes of reaction, in the face of the etiologic agents of disease. This material environment is determined by wages, nutrition, housing, clothing, culture and additional concrete conditions and historical factors ....
>
> Waitzkin 1981, p. 93

A broad perspective was presented from findings through observations of the working classes in England. A range of conditions are cited. Waitzkin presents these issues as somewhat of a stark reminder of the not too distant past and where the roots of sickness lay – in poverty and social deprivation. The workplace was an area of exploitation of men, women and children. Social organisation of the period ensured a reinforcement of such conditions across the private and public divide.

He makes clear that medical intervention and public health education initiatives are vital in social change, but at the same time underlines the necessity for political will. Policies that emphasise social action, wealth redistribution and combined education, as well as giving people a stake in society were regarded as necessary for health improvement.

> ... A healthy population was a worthy goal in its own right, but also for the sake of national development. The country's productivity suffered because of workers' illness and early death. Yet improving the health of workers was impossible without fundamental structural changes ....
>
> Waitzkin 1981, p. 96

When applied to the workplace, health programmes, for Waitzkin, cannot prosper without altering the illness generating conditions of the workplace. The elements in his thesis refers to:

1   economic production very much along the same path as Engels, Marx and Navarro.

> ... The organisation and process of production ... [where] disease and death ... developed directly from exposure to dusts, chemicals, time pressures, bodily posture, visual demands and related difficulties that workers faced in their jobs. Environmental pollution, bad housing, alcoholism, and malnutrition also contributed to the poor health of working class people, but on balance these factors mainly reflected or exacerbated the structural contradictions of production itself ....
>
> Waitzkin 1981, p. 97

2 inequalities in the distribution and consumption of social resources and their impact on people in society. Health problems emanated from poverty, malnutrition, linguistic inefficiency and the poor education reflected in the type of work people were able to obtain if at all (Virchow 1957).

3 class structure, underdevelopment and the impact of imperialism. For example, Allende discusses the conflicting role of medicine inherent in the class structure and that very structure being responsible for some of the health problems that existed amongst the working populations, largely as a result of exploitation.

The emphasis rested on issues connected to reform in a political context to improve the working conditions of people. At the same time, the ideas begin the process for later works in terms of analysing the inequality perspectives within the workplace affecting other groups including women and ethnic minorities.

Criticism

The major criticism of his work is that he does not go far enough in terms of developments in a neo-Fordist era and the impact on working groups, i.e. holding professional and administrative status in the workplace. Neither does he use the thesis to either encourage or expel the myth of meritocracy and the processes brought into play to withhold resources and inhibit the worker's progress. However, granted, his explanations focus on specific historical periods and the notion of work in manufacturing industries. Further analysis is required in light of new technologies. The role of women at work also requires further development.

Psychosocial approach

Bertil Gardell

Bertil Gardell was born around the late 1920s and died aged 59 in 1987. He was Professor in the Department of Psychology at the University of Stockholm, Sweden.

Gardell worked with many people throughout his life, mainly in a researcher capacity, and was firmly of the belief that working people had the capacity to conceptualise, change and ultimately control the nature of their own working life. Over a 25 year period, Gardell made a substantial contribution to the field of psychosocial work environment research. His work spans several disciplines: epidemiology, health policy, historical sociology, organisational sociology and psychobiology. However, his major preoccupation rested with the impact of the *work process* and *orga-*

nisation on physical and mental health. Although the field of study now extends to Australia, north and south America and western Europe, many researchers and practitioners consider Gardell's influence in this field.

Collectively, Gardell published some 130 books, chapters, reports and articles during the period 1963–1988. His major publications include: *Technology, Alienation and Mental Health*(1971), his PhD thesis; *Job Content and the Quality of Life* (1976); *Assembly-line Health Care. A Research Project on the Organisation of Care and Work in Hospital* (1979), with Rolf A. Gustafsson; *Codetermination and Autonomy: A Local Trade Union Strategy for Democracy at the Workplace* (1981), with Lennart Svensson.

For Gardell, work is one of the most important sources of social and psychological well being in that it provides much of the meaning and structure to adult life.

Gardell was involved in practical work reform and change efforts during the 1950s and 1960s. Gardell's point of departure from the historico-political thesis espoused by Navarro is to take on *the problem of work organisation* and *alienation* as a more manageable concept; Gardell set out to demonstrate its impact on the individual at work.

In the 1960s, Gardell returned to academia to conduct a series of studies to explore the concept of alienation and mental health. Operating at both an empirical and a political level, Gardell, together with his colleagues, studied a series of work settings and found that deskilling, loss of freedom, passivity, social isolation, and related aspects of alienation had an impact, not just on psychological, but on physiological functioning (Frankenhauser 1986).

Along with his colleagues, Gardell found, for example, that work which socialises people to be passive on the job carries over into non-working life. A phenomenon that he investigated in Sweden – one which deserves greater consideration – was that those who have little control over their jobs continue to be passive in other aspects of their life as well.

Alienation at work contributes to larger political and social alienation. By contrast, workers with a greater degree of self determination and control in their work demonstrate greater interest and involvement in addressing and changing the problems they encounter in their workplace ....

Johnson et al. 1991, p. 9

Gardell also provided a useful counterpoint to the idea that it is psychologically demanding work that is uniquely deleterious to the body and the psyche. His observations point to the importance of boredom, dehumanisation, and the other host of small dissolutions that occur.

In *Alienation and Mental Health* (1971) he laid the foundation and ideological position for his work in years to come. Although largely Marxian in tradition, his focus centred on the workplace and the industrial production system. Although ownership was acknowledged in part to be an issue, as originally espoused by Marx, it is not one that Gardell wished to take on board, although current reading suggested the evidence for making such a decision is partial. The finding in his previous research (Gardell and Dahlstrom 1966) rather suggested that the problem of alienation emanated from authoritarian leadership, fragmented and constrained work within traditional industrial environments. In other words, the labour process and management systems were, for Gardell, the major contributory factors to alienation.

One, however, needs to take account of the historical context in which this work was placed in terms of work and work tradition (1960s and 1970s Europe). The issues are similar to those marked out by Braverman (1974).

In *Labour and Monopoly Capital*, Braverman renewed interest in Marx's concern relating to social conflict and control in the labour process. His focus was on the structurally determined imperatives of managerial control, its effects upon the workers, and the dynamic process of degradation and deskilling that occurred on the shop floor. These elements were demonstrated prior to the impact of alienation on the individual in the workplace. However, the essence of this process is brought into sharp focus by Blauner (1964).

Gardell's early influence came through Blauner's *Alienation and Freedom* which is utilised to inform aspects of his work. It is through Blauner, that Gardell locates his tools for measuring the extent of alienation experienced within different work environments. For Blauner, alienation existed when workers were not able to take control over their immediate work process, unable to develop a sense of purpose and sense of identity with integrated industrial communities. The ability for personal expression was also retarded. This was demonstrated in meaninglessness, powerlessness, isolation and self estrangement. Technological factors, such as design of the manufacturing process, content and organisation of work, for the most part, determine the attitudes of the individual at the workplace.

The work process had an impact on the psychological needs of people and issues such as:

1   the need for personal say; personal control
2   need for interesting and meaningful work
3   the individual's participation in the firm as a social system would assist in maintaining health and harmony at work.

Self esteem is seen as a necessary component of worker health:

> ... we proceed from the concept of self esteem, which is central not only to our principal criteria of work satisfaction but also to theories of positive mental health ... we postulate that self esteem is strongly rooted in work for most people in our society.
>
> Gardell 1971, p. 149

Those qualities which undermine self esteem, as stated also by Blauner and Braverman, could lead to detrimental effects related to prestige, ability and general satisfaction in life. These ideas were also found in the works of Friedlander (1966), Forslin (1969), French and Kahn 1962 and Kornhauser (1965).

Personal say, personal control

Gardell was writing at this point about the manufacturing industries with fragmentation of work processes and rapid increase in technology. The issue of personal say/personal control relate to the ability to influence corporate policy, negotiate aspects, terms and conditions of employment, and immediate control over the work process.

> 1 the individual's personal control over his own working pace and rhythm
> 2 the individual's scope for regulating the pressure to which he is subject
> 3 the individual's personal control over physical motions, breaks and the like
> 4 the individual's scope for influencing production quantitatively and qualitatively
> 5 the individual's scope for selecting methods and tools to perform a task
>
> Gardell 1965, p. 15

This is extended in the process and execution of work:
For Gardell, these aspects of work assisted in determining the individual's sense of autonomy and awareness of constraint and stress on the job.

Need for interesting and meaningful work

Gardell looked closely at the Taylorist process in work (as did Blauner and Braverman) to gain a sense of development of the individual. He noted that scientific management caused a considerable amount of fragmentation and specialisation of tasks, and hence the individual saw less and less of their contribution to the whole. Hence, to gain meaningfulness in work, the individual's relationship with the product, organisation of the work process and particular skills need to be considered.

This extended the work of Marx in his ideas on the division of labour which impacted on the productive process and produced an instrumental workforce (Grint 1998).

The impact of boredom, monotony and the lack of skill discretion later explored by Marmot and Theorell (1984, 1986, 1987), was found to impact on cardiovascular disease predisposition in civil servants. The issue of meaninglessness became equally applicable to the service sector and professional occupations as earlier manufacturing (Frankenhauser 1989). Gardell's influence provided the precursor for further development in investigations into workplace health.

The Individual's participation in the firm as a social system

Marx's view of the market economy and commodity exchange saw every worker (or productive group undertaking mindless repetitive tasks) turning into competitors, setting individual against individual, reducing the capacity for social relations in the workplace. Again, Gardell related these principles to administrative and technological structures to develop his approach. The issue of social isolation arose when the worker was not able to gain any enthusiasm or affinity or identity from the workplace. This was also the case in situations of limited contact, especially in compensation for the limited control the worker may have over work.

The issue of isolation for Gardell was the:

1 perception of not being in touch with people and not entering into a fellowship of any kind (estrangement)
2 perception of not belonging to and feeling affinity with a group (group homelessness)
3 perception of not accepting the standards and goals which apply in the job world (anomie).

Gardell 1971, p. 153

He outlined why work could lead to alienation and its impact on the individual. The most noted type, the passive nature, was the result of a depreciation in the value of the work performed by the individual which was only seen as a means to an end. It paid a wage and no more. The work was not perceived to be engaging.

For Gardell, the process of production, its organisation, its workings, its function and ability/inability to meet the satisfaction needs of others were the aspects of alienation. This was a point of departure from Blauner's work which expressed alienation in terms of job performance and turnover in relation to technology.

Gardell and his colleagues developed a series of studies on alienation and mental health in a variety of work settings. They found deskilling, loss of freedom, passivity, social isolation and related aspects of alienation had their impact on the psychological and physiological functioning of workers. His studies also led him to discover that work which socialises the individual to be passive, also carried through into other spheres of life.

During his early studies, Gardell began to examine aspects of the individual worker and the psychosocial environment which might serve to explain the differences observed in stress responses and disease rates within the working population. Two approaches have developed from his findings. Firstly, the individual worker's predispositions, attributes, and skills – an orientation that might be considered congruent with the political and cultural values that predominate in the United States. Secondly, European researchers, particularly of Norway and Sweden, emphasise the structural characteristics of the work setting itself, and have focused their attention on the resources available to individuals or groups to meet demands for production and performance.

The centrality of the *concept of control* in the work environment field is to a significant degree one of the legacies of the research of Gardell. In *Alienation and Mental Health* (1971), he compared different types of production systems in terms of the major psychosocial determinants of mental health status. He hypothesised that rationalised forms of production come into conflict with fundamental needs of self esteem, such as the ability to maintain influence and control over one's work situation.

Gardell generally observes work in industrial production systems as designed sometimes to be incompatible with a broadened concept of health and safety as well as the social goals of democratic working life. In connection with technology and organisation design, lack of control of pace and working methods severely impoverished job content and socially isolated jobs. These conditions lead to both physiological and psychological stress which manifest in differing signs of ill health. Also, people cope with these conditions by non-participation and by holding back human resources.

Gardell saw workers as *subjects* able to respond to their environment, and acted formally and informally to alter it. His role as researcher was to operate in concert with working people to examine, and ultimately change the nature of the work process. He was a staunch believer in equality and fairness. Through a number of empirical studies, Gardell consistently found that if workers have some degree of control over their work situation, they seem to fare better in a number of different respects.

Control in turn, can be said to be constituted of three main dimensions:

1 the freedom to make decisions;
2 competence or knowledge which enables the worker to use this freedom;
3 contact with fellow workers, which enables the worker to co-ordinate activities in relation to others and to develop joint learning processes, relationships of social support and so forth.

Gardell had developed this view on the basis of empirical investigations with a naturalistic foundation. The successive emergence of the idea of control brought a major step further towards Karasek's concept of the demand-control model, did, however, imply a change in the theory of science implicit in Gardell's work.

Control equals activity. It is equal to activity between different courses of action to meet workplace problems. When the possibility of worker action was brought into focus, the worker changes from being an object to becoming a subject, someone whose actions shapes his or her own fate.

Problem with the notion of control

1 Gardell saw one of the main tasks of people was to uncover *social laws*, ways of acting within particular settings. It is assumed that Gardell implied group process and culture within organisations (although it appears that culture was not entirely made explicit in his work seen to date). However, such 'laws' can alter because those people under the control of a 'leader' can also change the rules, so the existence of true laws may be a problem or confined to an elite group who encourage/ coerce others to conform. Even those who are controlled by others, can alter their behaviour as a reaction to their 'controller' deliberately to create chaos as a negative response to being controlled.
2 To see the worker operating as an agent can, under certain circumstances, undermine welfare policy since it can locate the onus of responsibility on the worker.

The important foundations in Gardell's position in the study of workplace health lay in social isolation (Gardell 1979; Gardell and Gustavsen 1980). The perspective observes man's capacity at work and the connection to physical fitness. Taylorism looked at the limitations of man's capacity and the extent to which such limitations could improve productivity. For the most part the capacity rested with the physiological in terms of ergonomic and climatic impact, whilst the psychological was largely neglected. According to the limited range in which psychology was employed, it was in 'finding the right man for the right job'. (Gardell 1981, p. 4; also see Chapter 4).

Observing of Scandinavian life in the 1950s, Gardell attempted to link ideas relating to human relations and scientific management theories and the Welfare State. Antagonism to such ideas began to emerge in the 1960s, especially in relation to issues of specialisation and control in the workplace, in the sense that it was likely to have an impact on human and social relations. One response to this speculation came in Lysgaard's study on workers collectivity (Lysgaard 1960). Gardell drew on his notion of control and collectivity to drive the importance of social relations at work.

Starting with the informal relationships between workers as accounted in the Hawthorne studies (Roethlisberger and Dickson 1950), Lysgaard extended these and found that the workers' need protection against the demands of capitalism. Collectivity assisted in developing joint norms, drawing not only upon concrete experiences in the workplace but also upon general political ideas as founded in socialism. For Lysgaard, protection of the health of the workforce, through collective action within a democratic framework, was seen as the root to achieving better working conditions.

While Lysgaard's investigation was a case study, dedicated not least to model building, the 1960s also saw the emergence of a strong empirical tradition in Scandinavian work research, particularly in Sweden starting from conceivable conflicts between two systems of ideas. Drawing on Lysgaard's ideas, Gardell now saw that it had now been established beyond reasonable doubt that certain conditions such as deskilling have negative effects on workers.

Gardell extended further the notion of psychological capacities of humans through testing the impact of different types of work on individual groups of workers. More specifically, he looked at machine pacing of work rhythm and machine control of work methods.

He found that monotonous, repetitive work, activated only a limited part of total human capabilities. *Social isolation* was also an issue. The lack of possibilities for contact with others in jobs where piece-rates were introduced and the lack of opportunity for all workers to see the completed product, also took away the control over their creativity and pacing of the work. These systems were also seen to be detrimental to general physical capacity and the observance of safety.

Extension of the notion of social isolation and psychological stress through underdevelopment was applied to the *content of the job*, and the *extent of control* (Gardell and Gustavsen 1980). The lesser the content of the job, the less the worker has control over planning, design and methods employed in completing the work. The rewards are subsequently far fewer and have less meaning. This has an impact on the quality of life for many people as part of their identity is bound up with the work they do and their status. The health consequences, according to Gardell, are therefore accelerated and lead to physical and mental health problems as a result of dissatisfaction at the workplace. This was found to produce a rise in sleep problems, nervous disorders and intake of medication, especially as a consequence of increased psychosomatic problems. The monotony of particular types of employment were also seen to be a reflection of the worker's participation in social, political and cultural events. This is the antithesis for those workers who have far more rewarding employment.

The developments in Gardell's perspective very much equates with those offered as an extension of the original process of alienation in the works of Gorz and Marcuse (see Chapter 4).

Marianne Frankenhauser

Some of Gardell's founding works may also be linked to that of Marianne Frankenhauser, whose strand rests with job satisfaction and work stress. In other words the flip side of non-democratic hazardous working. In her work Frankenhauser rallied against ways in which individuals are focussed in the workplace to change, it is a point of departure from much of the work undertaken during the 1950s to the mid-1970s. Her work also moves from the medical model of health which also predominated at this time.

Frankenhauser warned that such interventions rest largely on individual behaviour change. Her approach to health improvement and health intervention connected with changing organisational structure:

> approaches involving changes at the structural level are much more controversial and complex than are changes at the level of the individual. The aim of [the] biopsychosocial approach to working life is to provide a broad scientific base for redesigning jobs and modifying work organisation in harmony with human needs, abilities and constraints.

Frankenhauser's work begins with a position similar to Gardell, but made a deeper exploration of the dimensions detrimental to health caused by certain components in the workplace.

Gardell provided a theory for positive working whilst Frankenhauser (1986) provided the evidence which culminated in poor worker relations. In *A Psychobiological Framework for Research on Human Stress and Coping*, she makes use of some of the elements originally identified in Gardell's *Alienation and Mental Health* (1971), namely understimulation and control, and develops points of departure specifically in her work with women and the notion of unwinding and the connection with leisure.

Issues of understimulation

When work demands are repetitive, the human brain becomes undernourished. The performance also deteriorates if the person's skills are underutilised. Stress, in this case becomes a threat to health and safety. In her observations of the Volvo plant in Sweden, Frankenhauser saw that under-stimulation and opportunities for socialisation were the key risks to health in the workplace. From her observations of workers in the control room, she found that where the process of monitoring, a vital aspect of their work, meant the difference between positive or disastrous economic consequences: 'In a monotonous environment the ability to detect signals starts to decline in less than half an hour. Yet the job calls for unfailing attentiveness and preparedness ...'. (Frankenhauser 1985).

Lack of stimulation through work forces workers to seek stimulation elsewhere but can have the effect upon general constriction and confinement in general activity (see Chapter 1 re: issues of boredom).

Frankenhauser focussed on the office environment as a place where the process of deskilling is likely to be recognised. The computerised workplace is seen as portraying characteristics of a 'mental assembly line'. Some people had intellectually undemanding occupations where much of their time was spent feeding data into a computer. When compared to assembly line opera-tives, it was found that they displayed the same neuroendocrine stress profile, similar psychosomatic symptoms and sick leave.

The mental assembly line encourages focus on singular processes. The thought process is limited to thoughts of a singular dimension. The connec-tion with language, speech alongside behaviour pattern has yet to be estab-lished in research, although studies in activity deprivation have demonstrated child like behaviours in adults at work (Argyris 1964; Tennan et al. 1982; Lennerlof 1989).

Control

Like Gardell, Control over one's work, according to Frankenhauser, aids in the 'buffering' of stress symptoms by developing skills that enable an active, participatory work role, as well as finding greater job satisfaction and coping with problems at work.

The effect on the body in achieving positive and negative states is described in terms of hormonal secretion.

... the role of personal control in achieving a positive state has been demonstrated in a laboratory experiment in which subjects were exposed to performance demands in both low-control and high control situations. The low control situation induced effort and negative affect. Accordingly, adrenaline increased, but cortisol was suppressed. Simi-lar results were obtained in real life work situations differing with regard to the level of control.

Frankenhauser et al. 1980

The combinations of work overload and low capacity to make decisions also have a poor impact on the cardiovascular system. This is not the case if the workload is high and the decision latitude is also high.

Unwinding: the work/leisure relationship

Women, for the most part, are considered in Frankenhauser's studies, especially in relation to work in the private and public domain. In promoting health, this is an important factor when observing health problems in women who work and have the added responsibility of home and family.

Unwinding is a key concept in health promotion, and the most important obstacle to unwinding after work is the 'second job', which a large part of the employees take up when they return home, i.e. demands related to the family, children, household, and a number of home management duties.

Frankenhauser 1989

The concept of the *total workload* introduced by Frankenhauser, enabled the measurement of the workload in paid work and other variables which impinged on stress/ability to unwind.

The total workload concept communicated the total working day and took on a fuller definition of what was considered to be work, encompassing the notion that work that also has physiological and psychological consequences when related to stress, but that is also unpaid. This implied work is carried out in the public and private domain. Frankenhauser's studies largely rested on whether or not women managers were inclined to experience more persistent stress as a result of fewer opportunities to unwind because of their domestic chores and child rearing. Males and females were included in the study. Her conclusions were not surprising. Women managers had their blood pressure, heart rate, self report notes on daily activity, and catecholamine secretions assessed. It was found that these women demonstrated no signs of unwinding during the evenings. Their noradrenalin levels also continued to rise on arrival at home after work, whereas many men with similar jobs noradrenalin levels fell markedly after 5 pm, the end of their working day. Frankenhauser concluded that unwinding after work was a male privilege.

Frankenhauser's ideas provide a useful point of departure for study within all areas defined as workplace. The sustained impact on women in these roles have yet to come to fruition in research, as well as issues relating to lone parents, male lone parents and ethnic groups with similar workloads in the public domain. Issues of racism as well as domestic situations have not yet been located in her research.

Ellen M. Hall

Hall follows Frankenhauser's connection between the private and public domain and impact on the individual in the observation of stress. Progress since the 1970s brand of feminism in the western world for Hall brought its limitations in the way health issues were studied for women. Women were studied primarily if their contributions were relevant in terms of difference to men, especially strength and endurance, or in their reproductive capacities.

Additionally, investigations of women's working lives have been used in deeply contradictory ways:

1   to argue for protection
2   to suggest that the workplace should treat every employee fairly
3   to campaign for more and better child care (Skrzycki 1988)

Hall begins with the premise that much work undertaken regarding the health of women and work is rather limited, especially in the field of stress. The exceptions have being those performed by Haynes (1980), La Croix (1984, 1987), Feinleib and Kannel (1980) who have used the Framingham Heart Study to evaluate the impact of women's work on cardiovascular disease. Although other researchers have looked at mixed and female population, the Framingham data represented a major study in terms of health outcome. The study compared employed women with housewives and have found that there is more type A behaviour, more daily stress, and more marital dissatisfaction in employed women than in housewives.

However, housewives and working women were found to have the same incidence of coronary heart disease (CHD). In comparing white collar professionals with blue collar workers, no elevation in risk was observed. The occupation at greatest risk was found to be female clerical workers with major domestic responsibilities and a punitive or restrictive psychological work environment. The facets of home and work that were associated with higher rates of CHD were decreased job mobility, repressed hostility, and having the combination of a non-supportive boss, children, and a blue-collar husband. None of the usual risk factors (smoking, age, blood pressure, serum cholesterol) were associated with CHD in these clerical workers. In short, several studies that are specifically concerned with the physical health of working women indicate that working does not appear to be in and of itself harmful to women.

In her studies relating to control in the work environment and stress in the workplace in Sweden, she formulated the following conclusions:

1   Sex segregation in specific forms of work was generally commonplace, therefore, work is the place where most people are socialised with and by members of their own sex. The topic of adult socialisation in terms of impact on men and women by the same sex has yet to be explored in detail.

2   Women have fewer occupations, of a less diverse character from which to choose than do men. Career options are still limited for women.

Although her position is not as developed as Frankenhauser, she provides some useful food for thought in terms of development in the study of health, work and women.

Political reform approach

The trades unions

At the end of the nineteenth century some momentum had gathered relating to the health, but predominantly safety needs of the worker. The Workmen's Compensation Act of 1897 became an important piece of legislation which considered the issue of accidents at work (it wasn't followed up until 1960 with an act covering diseases). However, the primary purpose of this legislation was not to care for workers, or to prevent accidents and diseases, but to assist employers rebut claims for damages. For this, company doctors were increasingly employed, which heralded an unhappy introduction of medicine to industry.

When the 1897 Act was first introduced, workers were owed compensation irrespective of negligence. The unions' position was to rely not on legislation but on the judicial system to prove negligence in the courts. This strengthened their position with the workforce because it brought into sharp focus specific employment practices which amounted to dangers to the health of a vulnerable workforce.

The mining and pottery industries, for example, led the way in terms of investigations in occupational hazards and was soon followed by the munitions industries. Safety issues became a feature of such enquiries.

The Whitley Report (1919) was advocating the idea and reality of joint employers and workers councils operating alongside the Factory Inspectorate.

During the 1920s the objects of the TUC at that time contained no special reference to accident prevention although as time progressed it became a useful lever to drive reform. The nearest the stated objects came to this matter was in these terms:

2(a) ... To promote the interests of all its affiliated organisations and generally to improve the economic and social conditions of the worker.
(b) In furtherance of these objects, the General Council shall endeavour to establish the following measures....
(6) Industrial accidents and diseases. Adequate maintenance and compensation in respect of all forms of industrial accident and disease.

Subsequently the objects were changed to their present form:

2(a) To do anything to promote the interests of all or any of its affiliated organisations or anything beneficial to the interests of past and present individual members of such organisations ....
In pursuance of such objects the Congress may do or authorise to be done all such acts and things as it considers necessary ... and in particular shall endeavour to establish the following measures and such other as any Annual Congress may approve ....
(Item 6) Occupational accidents and diseases. Adequate maintenance and compensation in respect of all forms of industrial accidents and diseases. The promotion of legal standards of health, hygiene and welfare in all places of employment.

Williams 1961

In 1924, The TUC publication, *The Waste of Capitalism*, made it absolutely clear that workers should be involved in the decision making processes of their own working environment.

This challenged the value of joint negotiating committees where workers had little power. The publication encouraged workers to be conscious of their working conditions and to ensure employers were left in no doubt if this was less than satisfactory.

Participation in union activity during the 1920s and 1930s reduced following the General Strike and mass unemployment in Britain, yet at the same time increased bureaucracy in leadership. It was this leadership that embraced preventive health and safety. Fear of unemployment, saw hazard pay and compensation for workers come on to the Trade Union agenda and became the means of visible attack on employers for continuing to foster dangerous working conditions.

The late John Williams' work, *Accidents and Ill health at Work*, emphasised that for all the efforts of the trade union, there really had been little change during this period. He found that one in every 15 working people could be expected to be injured in some kind of industrial accident each year, the Factory Inspectorate was understaffed and demoralised, the average fine for breaking the Factories Act was £14 (it was £8 in 1938) and that voluntary organisations, compensation, research and safety committees were all ineffective in reducing this workplace carnage.

He concluded:

> The outstanding features of the British system are that its growth over 150 years has been piecemeal, uncoordinated, anomalous and limited .... Another remarkable feature is the limited scope given to workmen who run the risks of industrial injury to take part in establishing safe standards at the workplace.
>
> Williams 1961, p. 31

There were, however, missed opportunities, especially regarding white lead (1934) and cadmium poisoning which did not resurface until the 1950s (see Chapter 3).

Beta-naphthylanine was recognised by Imperial Chemical Industries to be a major contributory factor in the development of bladder cancer, especially amongst rubber workers, but they continued to make it. Fines were eventually imposed but, PVC (another carcinogen) manufacture continued without due attention to health impact, hence the same mistakes were repeated.

Medical advisory issues at work began with Thomas Legge. When he died in 1956, Dr. H.B. Morgan took over. The TUC under Morgan saw the extension of provisions for medical advice and service to affiliated unions.

The basic attack of the movement had now developed into four avenues:

1   improvements in the accident compensation system
2   improvement of existing statutory standards
3   extension of statutory standards to new fields
4   the exploitation of joint machinery with employers and Government Departments for these purposes

Momentum grew in the interest of health and safety issues as a result of research under the auspices of the MRC during the 1950s. It was an issue that the unions could continue to agitate for governmental attention, with growing evidence of ill health caused by toxic materials, pollution and unsafe practices. Union membership increased during this time and TUC conferences continued to give health and safety issues a greater profile. By 1954, a motion was forwarded urging the government to action accident prevention measures in every type of working environment, factory or office, by the introduction of joint committees. There were still obstacles to be overcome even with repeated requests during 1956 and 1958 as the motion was not carried: the General Council argued that it might see a reduction in the employers' liability in the event of accidents. All the unions were able to achieve was improvements in existing legislation. Some individual unions were able to gain in the foundries and mines, but as a collective, there was still no unified success in formulation policy in health and safety.

The 1959 TUC at Blackpool received a General Council report which included the results of the comprehensive review of the provisions of the

Factories Acts. This is a most valuable review; but whilst appreciating this, it must be remembered that it represents only part of the problem in relation to the requirements of a comprehensive accident and ill health prevention service. The review, presented in the form of a memorandum to the government, dealt with a number of important points including the following:

1   the need for more factory inspectors;
2   the need for more factory inspections and for the ultimate aim of inspection at every workplace once each year;
3   more attention and financial provision for research into safety and health problems;
4   the need for a comprehensive occupational health service;
5   more attention to the problems of older buildings and substandard conditions in older workplaces;
6   more attention to problems of temperature and ventilation;
7   more power for factory inspectors in specifying safety requirements;
8   improvement in existing standards as to

    (a) ladders
    (b) weight-lifting
    (c) eye protection
    (d) provision of safety footwear

9   compulsory notification of dermatitis.

In reaffirming the TUC attitude to the importance of joint safety committees in the formulation and implementation of safety policy, the report merely emphasised the significance of the current review of the safety committee position being conducted by the Industrial Safety Advisory Committee; but at the same time it repeated the opinion that a uniform programme for safety committees was not practicable.

It was the build up in the Robens' enquiry that fired up the unions' position to build evidence, a total of 600 pages, so some way towards health and safety legislation was carved out. The evidence was a joint effort between the TUC, CBI, industrial associations and government department. Despite this, Robens still concluded that the main issue relating to accidents and ill health at work was apathy (Clutterbuck 1980). The tensions and conflicts between profit and health protection and health improvement continued despite legislation in Health and Safety during 1974. However, the unions, along with support from the Work Hazards groups, have continued to form a useful function in monitoring health problems, intelligence gathering and maintaining pressure on employers to improve standards in the workplace (see Chapters 2 and 3).

Bertil Gardell

Gardell perceived the following aspects of work to have an adverse consequence on the effectiveness of the individual worker:

- machine pacing of work rhythm and machine control of work methods
- monotonous repetitive work, activating only a limited part of total human capabilities
- lack of possibilities for contract with other people as part of the ongoing work
- piece rates and related payment systems, which in addition to contributing to employee wear and tear, are often detrimental to the observance of safety requirements
- authoritarian and detailed control of the individual be it through foremen or impersonal systems (computer based planning)

The issue of *technological determinism* is addressed in terms of work reform strategies. Gardell perceived this issue to be grossly exaggerated to the extent that work organisation had become specialised beyond what was seen to be necessary. It became apparent that a change in the individual's work situation was paramount to adjustment in social and human problems in working life. Experience in the work of Scandinavian researchers provided support to the notion that the organisation of work should be based on production groups and not on individuals. There was emphasis on the need to provide workers with the capacity to plan and perform work that is within their range and that extended their individual abilities. It was suggested that the element of control should also be established in this frame of thought.

> Foremen and technical experts should be geared to the needs and demands of the production groups – as resources for these groups – and not to functional requirements specified by higher organisational levels. A work organisation which has such production groups as its primary building blocks seems to have the potential for counteracting problems of fragmentation and coercion; among other things owing to the following properties of the group. In a group context the individual can expend his or her possibilities for attaining some degree of freedom and competence through work. Opportunities for learning and variation in work will be improved. The individual and the group will be able to achieve improved control over the rhythm and methods of work. Opportunities for contact and solidarity between people will be improved.
>
> Gardell 1977, pp. 8–9

The approach linking greater co-operation on the shop floor does have its limitations. The field experiments undertaken in Scandinavia during the

1960s demonstrated some of these issues. In Norway, the Industrial democracy programme emerged as a collaborative scheme between Working Life Researchers, Employers Confederation and the Federation of Trade Unions.

The programme involved a series of phases. The first was concerned with testing new forms of work organisation of the time at selected areas of work. The second phase involved communicating and publicising the experiences in the areas of experiment. The same activity was undertaken in Sweden but with a much reduced profile.

The Norwegian project underwent a phase of hesitation following the initial stages of the project. *Working life* looked at the new ideas that had emerged, but did not readily commit itself to making changes. The reasons largely rested on structural issues of conservatism, issues of power and control in established positions within the workplace. The traditional practices of the trade unions also found some difficulty relating to the work researchers had undertaken, as they were perceived to be the ultimate guardians of worker's interests. However, the position they adopted was to sit on the fence and merely observe.

Gardell (1982) soon recognised the need for a *multi-level approach* to work reform. This would allow the unions to put their perspective forward and prevent the researchers from siding with management in terms of developing strategies for *organisational development*. The union position appeared to be emphasising some difficulty in establishing a reasonable relationship to such changes under the traditional legal situation, which provided managers with control over issues of work organisation. Further developments from the workforce would rest outside the sphere of statutory authority or obligation. This tended to be the position taken during the 1970s.

Much of Gardell's earlier research was performed and written during a time where precise rules in relation to health and safety were problematic in the sense that they tended to suit the views of the managers and owners of the work environment. They did not take the well being of employees into account. Not much attention was yet being paid to ergonomics or psychosocial loads in the workplace. This was underlined in the fact that problems in relation to health at work were not merely the result of a single factor. Indeed, this situation provided some illustration:

> ... as long as we stick to regulation through general rules, these interactions are rarely given the attention they deserve. Most general rules about loads and exposure limits are valid only if the factor in question appears in isolation. Work environment issues are turned into issues of measurement and the interpretation of measurement data, both of which require experts. The employees themselves have to sit passively on the sideline while their health and welfare are decided by others.
>
> Gardell 1973, p. 12

It was issues such as these that led to increasing pressure for legislative reform in Europe during the 1970s.

Gardell (1977) saw legislation to promote activity in terms of improving employee health as having one major advantage that people remained in gainful employment. The problem, however, rested on the ability to generate a legal–administrative strategy that could lead to the activation of the people in the workplaces without jeopardising their position. A subsequent link emerged between work environment and some of the issues of industrial democracy. Clarification of the issues in terms of problems experienced at work had to be established in order to move forward.

Gardell's position on health and safety legislative developments were highlighted in terms of the needs and priorities of employees:

> ... firstly, it is necessary to legitimise people's own experiences and definitions of the work environment problem; otherwise the employer can easily reject demands for improvements if he disagrees about what is problematical or about the suggested remedies. The employees easily become dependent upon experts to prove their case and if such experts are not available, or do, in fact, not argue the case of the workers, then issues are settled on the basis of management's authority.
>
> Gardell 1981, p. 14

For this reason, the legislation of this period expanded the rights of employees to influence the definition of specific issues. This was achieved through the establishment of safety stewards elected by the trade unions in all shops employing five or more people and the establishment of work environment committees in all workplaces employing over 50 people.

The second issue related to revision of priorities within the workplace.

> ... the new legislation has meant an upgrading of the priorities given to such issues as work environment, personnel matters and the like. We know, from various Scandinavian studies (Sind 1975; Qvale and Engelstad 1978) that matters like these are usually brought forth by employee representatives when they try to act on behalf of their constituency. The previous subordination of such issues to economic and technical goals, has been one of the hindrances from industrial democracy efforts.
>
> Gardell 1982, p. 14

Revision was necessary because work reforms had to be tailored to the individual needs of the workplace. Hence variations emerged in Norway and Sweden.

The link between the issue of job content on the one hand and general work environment issues on the other has been established somewhat differently in these countries. In Norway some of the basic conditions for employee activity are regulated in the Work Environment Act, particularly in section 12 ... the Swedish solution has been to have a less explicit regulation in the corresponding act; mainly by stressing the importance of work being arranged in such a way that the individual worker can influence his own work situation. Instead Sweden has passed an act dealing exclusively with the issue of employee participation on the local level as well as higher levels in the company.

Gardell 1982, p. 16

Democratic working

The Swedish position focused on the influence of the trade unions concerning the planning of work and the design of jobs and work organisation. The emphasis rested on tasks that could contribute to the development of skills and competence of the individual. Autonomous working groups are considered to be central to the democratic work organisation. There was emphasis on the group taking decisions relating to all issues within the work environment, process and practice.

As well as the process of work and the ways in which workers can participate socially and politically in the workplace, Gardell developed further views which are fundamental to health and health promotion within the work environment.

Although not formally acknowledged as health promotion activity until much later by fellow researchers such as Frankenhauser (1988), Gardell nonetheless sowed the seeds of organisational development where the worker is at the centre, and at the same time draws out those aspects of work process, worker relations and work environment that impact on health.

Their starting points began with the following premise:

Initially, workplace health and safety that would include psychosocial issues, had to have workplace action as a core element, only through activity would it be possible for the workers themselves to become subjects. Secondly, the use of inspectors, experts, researchers, however well meant, would only contribute to dependence and so lack of control that appeared to lie at the core of the problems of workers. Thirdly, to be able to set certain principles into a legislative framework, the context would need to include:

1   a broad obligation to operate within the field of health and safety on an enterprise level;
2   a broad right to raise work environment issues on the level of the enterprise and workplace;
3   the workers must have the right to participate in all phases and aspects of the work with work environment issues;
4   workers and management on the level of the enterprise must have a broad right to exercise their own judgement about definition of problems, setting of priorities and development of action plans;
5   public power should be applied to further local activity on health and safety issues in general rather than to focus only on the correction of specific work environment factors.

These ideas were not entirely new, and were found in older Norwegian legislation. However, although legislation denoted responsibility on the workplace, it gave the impression merely for reasons of principle. There was no explanation provided relating to the organisation of local efforts. Worker participation in workplace health and safety was largely limited to the right to elect safety delegates. If worker participation in the development of solutions to problems of health and safety is to take place, certain prerequisites must be fulfilled in terms of what type of work people have.

What did Gardell mean by worker participation?

The issue of worker participation was introduced to Gardell by the author Professor Hy Kornbluh of the Institute of Labour and Industrial Relations at the University of Michigan during the 1960s. The term *participatory work environment* encompassed both work environment and worker participation issues and focused on worker participation as a means of dealing with work environment problems.

In essence, it was a political goal. It was a means of debating and finding ways of dealing with poor working conditions. It encompassed a multilevel approach whereby workers formed the link with managers and trade unions to find suitable solutions to work based problems including health.

The role of trade unions was vital in this process. If they did not succeed in forming links then there was the danger of worker participation splitting into two separate parts. For example:

> ... one bureaucratic part based on legislation and collective bargaining that seeks to increase the influence for the trade union as an organization in economic life .... [The other aspect] dealing with worker participation at the shop floor level that concerns the ordinary worker in his daily activities.

In other words, collectivity was important in terms of formulating strategies and mobilising resources.

Was the participatory approach to work reform satisfactory?

Gardell was instrumental in the development of industrial work reform in Scandinavia in the late 1970s. His ideas centred on worker participation. This approach was seen as too much a break with tradition to be fully effective in legislation. Reform work therefore began in a mixed, conflicting legal and administrative fog. The same problems existed in Sweden and was less successful in penetrating Swedish work and health reforms.

The approach was ahead of its time, and clearly a threat to the traditional expert status. Enforceability was an issue. Although labour inspectors roles was to apply public power to compel local activity in health and safety issues it does not appear to have emerged. Independent power positions in directorates therefore were not easily controlled by ministries. Directorates also had boards with high level representation, e.g. labour market parties, and constitute independent policy centres. Health and safety in the 1970s had not much relevance in Norway or elsewhere. There was more credence attached to compensation for injury, and a limited willingness to contribute to strategies for dealing with health and safety issues. The service was at this time also largely underdeveloped.

Since 1982, many of the work environment issues have been integrated with issues pertaining to productivity and industrial democracy. Although the Act was not a great success, in that only 20 per cent in Norway implemented aspects over a 5 year period from 1977 to 1982, the psychosocial elements in relation to problems at work have been recognised as important.

The issue of co-determination was explored by Gardell and colleagues (Almex) in both formal and informal structures within the organisation. For example, the company had a health and safety committee with peripheral employees in majority and addressed issues concerning the work environment, machine acquisitions and rebuilding issues. Also, a finance committee and the board of the company became involved.

The groups met at between five and ten times a year. There were also informal networks through unions which channelled their views to shop stewards on health and safety committees.

Informal working groups developed their own rules regarding the rights and powers in decision making . Each group made decisions within its own sphere of competence, ensuring that they did not interfere or overlap with others. Supervisors were replaced by contact persons, who were elected members of each group. Supervision and internal distribution of work were decided by the group. Each group was responsible for training its members, facilitating job rotation, and the development of production methods. Technical experts were invited to provide support and assistance where needed. Where there were difficulties that could not be resolved by the group, then the local production manager or trade union representative would provide guidance.

The main features of a democratic work organisation are identified by Gardell as relating to autonomy. The group system is a collective work form based on equality of membership and entitlement. It was accepted that people have differences and that some produced more than others. There was no comparison made between individuals in this setting, and existing wage differences, according to Gardell, were to be abolished.

This would not necessarily be operative in many organisations in Britain by virtue of the past working environments history of class and hierarchy. The necessity for flexibility, networking and collectivity is now a feature, but salary/wage issues would continue to be a bone of contention, as well as knowledge and skills.

Gardell and colleagues recognised that they had an extremely difficult task to perform because the world of work was not yet attuned to the connection of psychosocial problems within the work environment. These problems were largely associated with semi-private problems and dealt with at individual level. They also felt that managers needed to recognise that they too are a causative element in these problems which is frequently ignored.

Although Gardell's work took him into the service sector (predominantly hospitals and transport), issues relating to the peculiarity of the organisation and its impact on the individual had not been fully developed. However, Vuori's (1982) perspective on human service sectors provided valuable insight into the mechanisms that are apparent. He developed the idea that health care is a form of production, and as such was open to the use of the same processes of production as other service or manufacturing industries. Patients were seen as raw materials, they triggered the production process of care, e.g. history taking, diagnosis, treatment, rehabilitation and follow-up (Dickens 1996).

Health promotion in organisations of the 1990s may be seen as a way forward in terms of fusing these efforts. It attempted to encourage negotiation within organisations and planning, as well as consultation at all levels within the organisation, whether it be to look at policy issues, to plan an event, the multisectoral/organisational approach can be seen as fulfilling that function of participation. There is an issue not yet fully explored about multi-site organisations, particularly in large service sectors such as hospitals.

The issue of health promotion also demonstrated participation that is largely voluntary, except where legal or statutory obligations come into force, e.g. nurses requiring moving and handling updating. Some dialogue is necessary in finding out the issues for the organisation, what workers want and how they negotiate problem solving in organisational development programmes, including health promotion. Making use of trade unions may be satisfactory, however, public service organisations are loyal also to their own professional bodies, so there is the tendency for workers to participate as professionals with existing knowledge to enable them to pursue their own health promotion initiatives by virtue of their standing as professionals having legitimate role within the organisation. This is separate from manufacturing where the division of labour is much more compartmentalised. However, the notion of hierarchy as related to participation in fields with a little changed management culture is a feature yet to be explored.

Gardell outlined that changes can be mobilised by workers themselves and not necessarily external agents. In the service sector, Dickens (1994) has pointed out that models and methods of human service quality have developed as a distinct entity from that of other service industries. The interaction between consumer and provider are crucial in human services and the description of and assessment of service quality by customer and provider must focus on the nature of this interaction.

Effectiveness for the company

The general consensus for Gardell's studies was that productivity did not decline. Looking beyond productivity, issues of effectiveness did emerge relating to the company's general goals, including quality and service, and its informal and flexible way of working. Therefore relationship arrived in factors such as product quality, initiative taking by the employees, customer service, capacity to meet deadlines and flexibility. During the study, managers noted generally that quality had not deteriorated as a result of autonomy. Flexibility had increased both within and between departments. Workers were generally more positive in their attitude to work.

Gardell drew some interesting conclusions from his experience at Almex which contributed to his thesis of the democratic working environment. These need to be explored within the context of the British work environment and also, perhaps transfer in discussions about professional groups and service industries.

The factors requiring greater consideration include:

1   union co-determination in decision making for company strategy;
2   groups for autonomous production;
3   resistance to unnecessary hierarchies and formal contact;
4   trade union education partly to build up knowledge but also to establish solidarity against elite recruitment and tendencies to push out non conformist workers;
5   active participation of all workers in the change process.

Gardell's position from this later work encouraged heavy union leadership in activating participation and gaining greater autonomy for the worker. This form of working has yet to be assessed in contexts where the work process serves different functions and different periods in time. For example, in the 1990s service sector where unions had far less influence in a workplace in Britain where flattened structures of management, and financial independence of some sectors, e.g. education, had been the norm since the late 1980s. The National Health Service had also changed as a result of policy reform in the drive towards greater efficiency and effectiveness. The 1990s advent of the purchaser provider split has increased competition within the service and hence is likely to be an unsuitable environment for democratic working. The issue had been more of survival than solidarity. New trust mergers with the most recent reforms have yet to yield a position in the sector. Autonomous working groups and issues of participation may appear in different guises, more perhaps on macro than micro political levels, e.g. devolution of the health sector in Britain.

This in time may be communicated in work process and influence within service organisations.

Some elements of Gardell's thinking can be taken into the sphere of workplace health promotion for further exploration. These can be linked with the components of the Ottawa Charter, namely:

- *Building healthy public policy* – health promotion policy combines diverse but complementary approaches including legislation, fiscal measures, taxation and *organisational change*. It is co-ordinated action that leads to health, income and social policies that foster greater equity. *Joint action* contributes to ensuring safer and healthier goods and services, healthier public services, and cleaner, more enjoyable environments (*which can be translated as active participation of the workforce*).
- *Creating supportive environments* – changing patterns of life, work and leisure have a significant impact on health. Work and leisure should be a source of health for people. The way society organise work should help create a healthy society. *Health promotion generates living and working conditions that are safe, stimulating, satisfying, satisfying and enjoyable (democratic working)*.
- *Strengthening community action* – at the heart of this process is the empowerment of communities, their ownership and control of their own endeavours and destinies. It draws on existing human and material resources in the community to enhance self help and social support, and to develop flexible systems for strengthening public participation and direction of health matters (*interaction with others, support each other, planning, participation, control*).
- *Developing personal skills* – health promotion supports personal and social development through providing information, education for health and enhancing life skills. By doing so, it increases the options available to people to exercise more control over their own health and over their environments, and to make choices conducive to health (*cooperation, control, skills, stimulation*).

These specific issues can be achieved within the work environment through health promotion but as yet they rest untested as we are unaware of what constitutes this phenomena at work, what it means to the workforce and those involved in facilitating the process.

There is one definition which has emanated from the Luxembourg declaration, but not yet articulated in any tested format (see Chapter 6). In other words researching this organisational phenomenon in light of the components which Gardell and colleagues spent some time carving out and providing a valuable link with the Ottawa Charter for health promotion, naturally, leads to the fact that the movement, although without formal name, had its origins in the workplace through the work of Gardell and his fellow scholars. Not only that but the essence of health promotion, although unqualified, emanated from the workplace as it pre-dates the work of Lalonde (Lalonde 1974).

It is a public policy phenomenon which has been translated into the workplace, whose peculiarities, characteristics, drive has not yet been made transparent.

Criticisms of Gardell's work reform

1   Gardell proposes that the autonomous group system is based on group work and collective responsibility. People are developing through their relations to others at a pace determined by themselves. One wonders if this actually produces a harmonious work environment or are people merely kept in their place? It assumes group ownership of ideas and responsibility. This may be useful in environments where products are produced, and even in some service sectors such as the police, but not in academic settings where there are a whole series of agendas. Not even in the NHS where resource as well as micro and macro political agendas come into play. This opens the issue of collectivity and its advantages and disadvantages in the workplace. Social skills systems of rewards and punishment, improvement in participation and control for the work, and subsequent impact on health in the workplace are too issues that requires further exploration.

2   Gardell also states that each member should be given the opportunity to learn all tasks within the group's working area. This increases flexibility, overview, and strengthens the group. At the same time, it makes work more intrinsically rewarding. Not sure about this. It can have the implication of no person's skills being indispensable. Again, it may be appropriate on the shop floor, but not in the professions, where abilities and skills are specialised, thus providing each 'expert' with greater autonomy over his/her own work. However, the issue of autonomy in some service sectors, particularly healthcare, education, medicine has seen a diminution in autonomy with the increase in quality control measures

including clinical governance. Surveillance has become a feature of the organisation in late twentieth century.

3   Gardell is also of the view that the group should not be allowed to recruit new members and replace workers without the consent of the union. The group should be encouraged to give shelter and support to members with social and other types of problems. But again, what if the group dislikes the new member. There is no explanation to support the view that new members may undoubtedly be placed in an awkward situation. The group may develop to be a rather constraining force – going against the creative expressionism and democratic working therefore curtailing any move towards health improvement.

Chapter 6

Workplace health promotion

Workplace health promotion (WHP) is not an easy subject to define when placed within the general context of health promotion/health education. Health promotion, and education for health continues to be an evolving and exciting subject for both practitioners and academics, and it is for this reason that any corollary to this will be faced with equal complexity.

Indeed there is identification with the view that many people working in the field have problems attempting to distinguish health promotion from health education (Wynne and Clarkin 1992). It is acknowledged that part of the problem also relates to a tension between some of the formal definitions of health promotion, which present an idealistic and comprehensive meaning, and the common practice of what is described as health promotion by practitioners in the field. This common practice also involves workplace health actions, for the most part directed at individuals in terms of attempting to achieve behavioural change, and which may be little more than disease prevention.

Workplace health promotion in the past was very much a laissez-faire matter. Any activities instigated were up to the forward thinking manager or interested group of employees following diet or exercise regimes during the lunch break or at the end of the working day. The effect of these activities were never evaluated in terms of the extent of behaviour change, improvement in well being or impact on the organisation in terms of reduction in sickness.

The effect and efforts of workplace health promotion in Britain particularly, greatly suffered from the health and safety ethos, and was rarely regarded as an important and separate area of health development. The climate now has somewhat altered with some employers experiencing claims made against their companies by their employees, for contracting smoking-related diseases, and suffering the adverse effects of stress (Wilkinson 1997).

Within the last few years, British employers have become more concerned with educating people about the reasons for ill health and helping them to adopt healthier lifestyles. Health promotion activity in the workplace has become extended beyond occupational health. It is concerned with utilising opportunities that a setting provides to promote healthy lifestyles, behaviour and attitudes in everyday life outside work (Taskforce 1993).

Others see workplace health promotion as a *multilevel* approach to health improvement (Gottlieb and McLeroy 1994; Shulz et al. 1995) or an *organisational approach* (Health Canada 1992; Wynne and Clarkin 1992; Grossman and Scala 1993) where both managers and employees have an equal responsibility for promoting health. Some specialists may also utilise the *business planning* approach to workplace health (Kizer 1987; HPW 1998) and there are those who operate the *democratico-participatory* approach (Svensson 1989).

Whilst therefore, it is difficult to be specific about the definition, workplace health promotion is becoming an area of increasing importance. There is too, accumulative recognition across the professions that it is an issue that affects them in the course of their activities. For example, occupational health nurses in broadening their remit (Pencak 1991; Pantry 1995), occupational therapists (see Jaffe 1986; Rider and White 1986) health educationists (see Nelson et al. 1987) and occupational physicians (see Feilding 1991; Green and Baker 1991; Schilling 1991) have all recognised the need for increased health promotion activity. More recently, the field of psychology, with the growing importance of stress at work (Cooper and Williams 1994) has also adopted some important notions of improving the health of the workforce.

During the 1970s, a number of American corporations and businesses introduced health promotion or 'wellness' programmes into the work environment. Worksite health promotion as it was known, was initially defined as a combination of educational, organisational and environmental activities designed to support behaviour conducive to the health of employees and their families (Parkinson 1982). In essence, workplace health promotion was seen to consist of health education, screening and intervention designed to change employee behaviour in a healthward direction and to reduce any associated risks to their health.

In some cases it was different from the traditional occupational health initiatives in that wellness programmes were interested in general health promotion, as opposed to a focus on health protection which concentrated on preventing occupational diseases or ensuring safe working conditions (Conrad 1987). There are however, other perspectives and they will become apparent in this chapter.

There has been an inclination for large companies to engage in health promotion activities. In the US, these have included Du Pont, Johnson and Johnson, Kimberley Clark and Coca-Cola. In the UK the movement has been gradual and has included the National Health Service, the Post Office, and the South Wales Constabulary. Activities have developed through various projects connected with the Health Education Authority and Health Promotion Wales and with support from the Confederation of British Industries (CBI) and the Trades Union Congress (TUC).

In other parts of Europe, workplace health promotion is developing gradually. The most successful strategies have involved mental health promotion. BKK in Germany has led the way in developing dual strategies for dealing with the alteration of the work environment as well as promoting health through individual behaviour change in what has come to be recognised as a more balanced approach to health promotion (Wynne 1994).

Definitions of WHP will become more apparent during the course of this chapter and are included alongside the emerging perspectives.

Emerging perspectives on workplace health promotion

Individual lifestyle and behavioural change

This perspective advocated by Jonathan Fielding, originally developed during the 1970s through studies of Canadian and US corporations. Others have adopted this perspective too in Britain. These positions are developed here.

For Feilding (1991), workplace health promotion emphasises a link between disease prevention and health promotion. He regards it as:

> ... Broadly subsuming both activities designed to assess and reduce future health risks and maximise individual health. The definition applies to some services delivered by usual providers of health care services, such as physicians, hospitals, and occupational medicine clinics, and services provided through organisations and individuals specifically providing non-medical assessment and counselling to maintain or improve health status through behavioural approaches (e.g. exercise, nutrition, counselling, stress management classes).

The definition reflects largely service provision in terms of practicality for those individuals in the workplace in need. The emphasis that the definitional issue is a complex one as it incorporates traditional knowledge relating to health protection, disease prevention and health promotion. For workplaces, however, they cannot be so easily separated because of the compulsory occupational medicine services, the emphasis on safety and accident prevention, as well as the necessity to provide information, counselling and screening for employees.

The driving factors relating to health promotion in workplaces relate largely to cost containment and reduction in insurance claims. Allied to this are the health issues that have arisen within the organisation, and thus some focus on these will at times be given priority over other issues. Feilding therefore provides the definition, although limited, which builds on traditional occupational medicine issues.

WHP for Feilding, was borne out of the employer's interest in reducing the excessive numbers of workplace injuries and health problems associated with hypertension. The employer sponsored activities consisted of emergency first aid programmes and CPR for all interested parties (Breslow and Feilding 1983). The essence of the initiation of such programmes rested on several factors:

1 recognition that the toll of the most common deadly diseases can be reduced through attention to lifestyle;
2 demonstration of the efficacy of both drug and non-drug treatment for high blood pressure;
3 development of effective behavioural medicine techniques to facilitate personal behaviour change; and
4 mounting employer costs of providing health benefits to employees.

Feilding 1984

Feilding developed this notion further following several years of research in the field. There were at least four interrelated strands in the development of WHP.

... Activities can be discerned
1 providing exercise facilities and hiring exercise physiologists to operate them;
2 addressing specific health problems, e.g. hypertension;
3 seeking to assess the overall health status of the workforce and developing programmes related to identified needs, e.g. taking advantage of the computerised health risk appraisals, available since the early 1980s, that both facilitated quantitative assessment of risks and harnessed the computer as a tool for health promotion management and evaluation; and
4 investing significantly in comprehensive health promotion programmes.
These activities started with careful planning and sought to integrate health assessments with efforts directed toward behavioural change for health and awareness concerning a broad range of personal health topics. Among large employers who developed comprehensive programmes in the late 1970s, and early 1980s were Kimberly Clark, Control Data Corp., Tenneco, AT&T and Johnson and Johnson

Breslow, Feilding et al. 1990, p. 14

In essence this is interpreted as firstly building on the traditional occupational medicine/health approaches of the US. Secondly, tackling head on health problems at work using the available resources. Also it is clear from Feilding's impression that we gain a sense that WHP was a rapid response to injury reduction and prevention. It is largely echoed in the medical model of health, specifically in relation to disease prevention through a focus on lifestyle and behavioural change. The issue of hypertension in the workplace was clearly a problem, hence the necessity to reduce the risk. Several studies undertaken in US corporations between 1967 and 1979 yielded the result that the elevated blood pressure was a firmly established risk factor to disease. This raised treatment in hypertension although the appropriate level above which drug treatment should be instituted remained controversial (Veterans Cooperative Administration 1967). Compared to other individuals at work, hypertensives develop approximately three times as much coronary heart disease, six times as much congestive heart failure, and seven times as many stokes (Veterans 1972). Lowering high blood pressure reduces the excess risk of hypertension-related morbidity and mortality in a dose-response fashion (Veterans 1970). Hypertension was found to be prevalent in workforce populations, with blood pressures in excess of 140/90 mm Hg found in 15 to 25 per cent of the worksite population (Veterans 1972). Employer sponsored hypertension detection and management programs have reported considerable success in identifying and controlling high blood pressure in employees. The introduction of CHD prevention programmes at the home office of the Massachusetts Mutual Life Insurance Company, saw the percentage of hypertensives under control increased from 36 to 82 per cent (National Heart, Lung and Blood Institute 1980).

As Fielding's perspective emerges from a specific healthcare tradition, it may be appropriate to pause and reflect upon that situation.

The US occupational health tradition

The US occupational health tradition was borne out of three main ideals. First the idea that prevention and control of hazards on the job could minimise and even eliminate risk, slowly replaced the opinion that accidents and diseases were unavoidable by-products of work. Second, the assumption by government for the health and safety of workers replaced the nineteenth century idea of laissez-faire, which had allowed for lack of significant social conscience pertaining to dangerous conditions of work, and minimal activity to protect men and women at work. The third and most recent change involved the idea that working men and women had the right to know about hazards on the job and to act to improve their own working conditions, including those related to job health and safety.

The continuous interplay between science and politics and the gap between awareness and action to eliminate hazards were two recurring themes in the US occupational health history (Karnell Corn 1992).

This traditional approach developed by Fielding and others, involves taking the opportunity to introduce health messages in the workplace, in as broad a means possible, to the lowest common denominator. This usually focuses on specific health messages in educating the individual to take more exercise, eat healthier meals and give up smoking. There is usually a planned programme of activity led by an enthusiastic member of the workforce or a health promoter with specific undertaking to lead such activity. Follow up information is usually provided by a member of the health professions in an advisory capacity with some supplementary literature. Focus is largely on the individual and has been widely criticised.

The focus rested on single health issues aimed at health related behaviours to reduce morbidity and mortality associated with coronary heart disease, strokes and cancers (Glasgow et al. 1995; Oldenburg et al. 1995). This approach has been adopted in part by some multinational corporations with a base in the US and companies in the UK (Feilding 1991; Wilkinson et al. 1998). The approach emphasises prevention making use of screening services and family planning clinics. Tactics involve education and counselling on a one-to-one basis or sharing experience with work colleagues, and is usually supplemented by basic popular literature on issues ranging from smoking, alcohol, exercise, sexual and mental health.

Advocates of workplace health improvement in the US believed that the nature of the job itself could lead to health problems, so their approach became based on prevention and health improvement. Interest in workplace health exploded onto the scene through employer sponsored activities to prevent disease and promote health which initially grew out of an interest in reducing the number of workplace injuries. Emergency first aid and cardio pulmonary resuscitation programmes were rapidly made available to employees (Feilding and Breslow 1983). This was also the case in Sweden with additional emphasis on product quality issues, where health problems were seen to interfere with the production process, having negative effect on the quality of products.

Workplace health activities commenced with careful planning and sought to integrate health assessments with efforts directed toward behavioural change for health awareness concerning a broad range of personal health topics.

The British position in workplace health promotion developed through a different set of circumstances. The late 1970 to early 1980s period saw interventions in worker health and well being generated from occupational health departments and *Look After Yourself* (LAY) and *Look After Your Heart* (LAYH) programmes. Health education was based very much on a 'sites' model and through government interventions in the early 1990s, the

Health of the Nation strategy has also contributed to this process. The process has been largely fragmented and adhoc. For the most part, the focus has been on policy development related largely to smoking or health issues raised by individuals during smoking cessation or stress management classes.

Health Promotion Wales, collaborating with Welsh employers such as the DVLA, Hyder (Welsh Water), Cefn Coed Hospital Swansea and the South Wales Constabulary has been the exception. With the assistance of the TUC and CBI, they have consolidated health promotion activity in the workplace through the *Make Health Your Business* awards. Each year, organisations are encouraged to enter the scheme to demonstrate both practically and through written evidence how they have addressed a variety of health promotion issues such as healthy eating, environmental care, smoking cessation and physical activity. The organisations making greatest efforts are presented with an award. The scheme has both improved health and brought good publicity to the participating companies. Currently, the most comprehensive approach to workplace health has employed corporate care strategies. To date, only a few companies have employed this holistic approach in the US (Betera 1990) and in Wales.

Although undoubtedly, workplace health promotion will, in the long term prove to be of considerable advantage to business, the benefits in some instances to date, have been perceived rather than systematically measured (Springett and Dugdill 1995). For the most part, the tendency in industry, has been to focus on medical screening. However, the difficulties run deeper than that and rest with a lack of infrastructure to monitor activity and provision of service. The other difficulty of course, lies with the perception of health promotion per se. This is developed further.

Britain's infrastructure

The success of workplace health promotion in Britain will rest largely on its infrastructure. Currently its development is in the hands of several disparate parties of health promotion officers, health promotion managers, environmental health officers (working largely with local county councils) or occupational health nurses. With all but a few exceptions, the majority of health promotion initiatives are in their early stages of development. The NHS has made its own contribution with the Health at Work project initiated by Simnett and Kemper, which has developed in the last few years; the effect has yet to be fully evaluated.

Much of the activity carried out is limited to the immediately perceived needs of the organisation and is usually negotiated within existing management structures. Occupational health nurses, in addition to the care and treatment tasks they perform, are usually able to initiate activities such as smoking cessation classes, employee screening and health fairs. This is largely initiated by themselves with some support from their managers.

Activities, however, in workplaces as a whole tend to vary. Firstly, there is a lack of finance for such initiatives, a major barrier for all but the largest enterprises. In the US, there is better provision as the majority cost is carried by the employer for health care. In most parts of Europe, the state is largely responsible for health care provision and thus militates against the development of more comprehensive health programmes (Wynne 1994).

A second obstacle relates to the general culture of health care in the UK. There is a tendency towards treatment and the emphasis on workplaces, often with good reason, is safety.

Thirdly, managers have a number of priorities for the service they deliver. That is to say, serving their customers, which means greater interest in productivity and meeting deadlines as opposed to health of the workforce. This is not to say that managers are complacent about worker health, it merely underlines the fact that the totality of the organisation and its function is far greater than the sum of individual health needs.

Fourthly, activity carried out in the workplace under the umbrella of health promotion is universally poorly evaluated. The benefits are not readily visible to the organisation, at least in the short term. Thus a tendency for one-off activity appears to be the norm. Allied to this argument, is the fact that health promotion officers will also need to build up a relationship with the organisation. Outsiders are naturally initially regarded with suspicion unless, of course, they have been invited in to perform a specific task (Wilkinson 1999).

The health promotion officer requires tenacity, patience and of course the ability to negotiate at a high level within many organisations and to persuade of the necessity for health promotion. A well established set of relationships with a number of organisations can be lost overnight if the officer moves to take up another post or her remit is altered by her paymaster who perceives different priorities for her in any financial year. This continuity has been increasingly difficult since the NHS reforms of the early 1990s where health promotion departments have become more fragmented as purchasers, provider or have an interest in both.

The fifth point relates to service provision. There are insufficient numbers of well trained people to deliver health promotion in the workplace. This has been particularly noted across Europe (Wynne and Clarkin 1992). Costs can also be prohibitive to pursue health initiatives, especially if greater intervention is required for a workforce with poorer health status. This point again cannot be fully proven as limited research exists in cost benefit assessments for health promotion (Cohen 1994; Haycox 1994).

Finally, evaluation. Once interventions in the workplace have been made, there are few studies which have effectively evaluated the impact on employee health or on productivity, whose methods can be drawn upon or further developed (Betera 1990; Wilkinson 1999).

Perception of health promotion in Britain

The traditional, yet pragmatic views of health promotion, even in some of the most enlightened organisations, have been the provision of healthy food choices in the canteen, the provision of leaflets and posters, and even perhaps a designated smoking area. Health promotion extends a great deal further. Many officers have been encouraged to deliver health promotion based on the perception of managers; the most likely reasons being time constraints and focussed priorities as a result of limited finance. Health promotion officers again in attempting to build relationships with companies, are put in this complex position of balancing poor perceptions and gaining entry, then gaining trust, noting uptake of say health fairs, and then if they are very lucky, the manager may want to maintain the momentum. This is when real health promoting activities can start to develop. Naturally, the process is a long one. Some officers never get beyond the health fair stage.

Occupational health services have also had an impact in the workplace and perhaps suggest an important link to workplace health promotion.

The link between health promotion and occupational health in Britain

The link between health promotion and the necessary provision of occupational health services is an important factor when considering how health promotion can be advanced. In 1973, the World Health Organization identified three major responsibilities of occupational health:

1   identifying and controlling known or suspected work factors that contribute to ill health;
2   educating management and workers to fulfil their responsibilities for health;
3   promoting health programmes not primarily concerned with work-related injury or disease.

The service has concentrated on and achieved most from the first two.

Indeed, it became recognised by the ILO Convention 161 (1985) on Occupational Health Services (OHS) that greater efforts were required to increase workplace health activity. In addition, this view was strengthened in 1987 by the WHO Expert Committee on Health Promotion in the Work Setting, that the workplace was changing and that pure concentration on hazards was considered to be not going far enough towards the drive to improve worker health (WHO 1988). However, the service has been somewhat constrained. Part of the difficulty lies with the position occupied by occupational health nurses in the sector and the numerous functions they are expected to employ.

The result has been that occupational health has become more focussed on safety, disease, risk prevention and care. Occupational health services are regarded as a secondary service provided by employers, in the interest of productivity, rather than wholly beneficial to the workforce. Thus, any time left for health promotion activity has been regarded with similar scepticism.

Health promotion was seen as an extension to the 'settings' work under the Health Education Council in the 1970s. Later *Health at Work in the NHS* and other similar initiatives in business have superseded this development.

As mentioned in an earlier chapter, occupational health is concerned with dealing with the effects of working conditions on employee health as well as employee health status and other health and safety needs at work. It encompasses many facets including setting up management systems to recognise ill health risks at work; identifying and controlling known or suspected hazards and risks to health in the workplace; providing first aid; helping employees with health problems to rehabilitate at work; developing policies to identify and deal with employees' problems which might impact on health and safety; and providing information, instruction and training on these matters to employees.

While both occupational safety and health, and workplace health promotion, seek to prevent work related illness and injury and promote employee health, the two fields have operated independently. Within a single firm, it is often the case that workplace health promotion interventions, and occupational safety and health (OSH), operate in isolation from one another. The intervention targets, personnel and methods are also dissimilar. Lifestyle, and safety are how both are distinctly regarded (Baker et al. 1996).

Workplace health promotion in organisations, serves as a convenient venue for health activity programmes, providing access to adult populations that might otherwise be difficult to reach. For the most part, the attempt to instil norms and values to facilitate successful individual behaviour change.

By contrast, OSH interventions attempt to reduce exposure to aspects of the workplace that are deleterious to employee health. OSH interventions may involve engineering strategies, e.g. making physical modifications to the workplace or work processes; or even administrative strategies including management initiatives that modify the work process or environment, and individual behaviour change strategies such as education and training to increase personal protective use (Goldenhar and Schulte 1994; O'Donnell and Harris 1994).

The basis for the difference in approach has arrived through historical roots, disciplinary background, and intervention ideology. In some cases, practitioners of these two approaches view each other as a competitor for resources rather than as partners working towards advancement in the field of employee health (Walsh et al. 1991).

Indeed, within the established model, both WHP and OSH programmes have faced challenges in developing considerable strategies for advancement that are effective to employee health. In some spheres, even the most conducive and well planned WHP interventions have not yielded the improvements in employee health behaviours (Glasgow et al. 1995; Sorensen et al. 1996). The same is true in OSH (Feildstein et al. 1993; Menzies et al. 1993). It is apparent that an alteration in the conceptual framework is necessary to bring WHP and OSH into a sphere where they can happily work in parallel to each other; and at the same time, clarify the role of the Workplace Health Co-ordinator or Workplace Health Promotion Officer.

Coverage of OSH and WHP programmes in Britain

Rantanen's review of occupational health services within the WHO European Region (covering 32 countries) estimated that only 44 per cent of workers within this region were covered by in-plan or occupational health services. A further 29 per cent of workers were covered by occupational health services linked to primary health care. Approximately 26 per cent have no service at all. The range of service provision within these countries is between 10 and 100 per cent (Ratanen 1991).

In the UK, the IFF Survey commissioned by the Health and Safety Executive (HSE 1976), showed that of organisations surveyed in the private and public sector: 8 per cent of the private sector workplaces use health professionals, primarily larger workplaces (32 per cent of those with 25 to 199 employees; 68 per cent of those with 200 plus employees). In the public sector 98 per cent of the workforce are employed in workplaces which use health professionals, and a higher proportion of those organisations use professionals with an occupational health qualification. Thirty six per cent of private sector employees and 53 per cent of all employees work in organisations using health professionals.

The US, by contrast, following its *National Survey of Worksite Health Promotion Activities*, revealed that over 65 per cent of US workplaces with 50 or more employees offered at least one disease prevention or health promotion activity for their employees each year (Meek 1993).

As mentioned above, occupational health personnel have had limited involvement in health promotion. This may in part be due to the specificity of medicine and treatment. It may also be due to models of occupational health adopted within the service.

Existing models of occupational health nursing do not allow for a problem solving approach or pose a challenge to established concepts (Fairburn and McGettigan 1994). The most recent approach to occupational health, however, has been utilising the Hansaari Model (Figure 1). This was launched by Ruth Alston in 1988 at Hansaari, Helsinki. It was initially utilised in the ENB training programme for occupational health nurses in 1990.

The Hansaari model is described as a outward proactive model encouraging nurses to raise awareness of their contribution to health issues in a broad environment. The Hansaari approach emphasises health promotion and sickness prevention (Friend 1990).

There is no fully co-ordinated and coherent strategy for workplace health promotion in Britain. For the most part, health authority or health trust employed health promotion officers did this as part of their remit. Occupational health nurses also, to a lesser extent, are encouraged to promote health in their work environment under the auspices of their employer.

However, there are other groups involved in workplace health activity which have evolved over recent years (Table 1).

The emphasis on lifestyle and behaviour change has also been predominant in the Britain and there are specific reasons for this. Firstly, few companies have comprehensive policies which focus on issues of work environment and management style, although awareness of the importance of these elements are increasing say, in no smoking policies and dealing with the adverse effects of stress. Secondly, the existence of what can only be recognised as a disunited occupational health service which is less than 30 years old. The service was difficult to establish, nurses have taken time to develop and become comfortable with their role, and the emphasis has been on health and safety matters as opposed to health promotion. Thirdly, the model of dominance in the health sector has been curative as opposed to preventive.

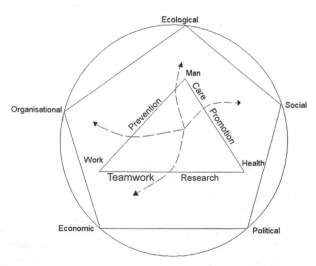

Figure 1   The Hansaari Model.

The breakthrough in health promotion is relatively recent, and workplace health promotion in the UK is still in its infancy. Fourthly, health promotion may not be a priority for the organisation as there are other pressing issues such as productivity.

Much consideration has been given to the development of WHP utilising general principles of health promotion. Subsequent measures for more accurate targeting of workplace health actions are being slowly implemented so that

1   they are applied across all groups of people in the workplace;
2   they can be directed at the underlying causes of ill health;
3   they combine diverse methods of approach;
4   they aim to make the worker more effective in terms of participation in the decision making process and general activity;
5   they broaden the perspective outwards from pure medical activity that includes working conditions and work organisations.

The British position in workplace health development stems from the occupational medicine tradition. Workplace health is still attempting to find its way in terms of whether it is distinct from the tradition or wants to operate in parallel or interlinked with occupational medicine.

Table 1   Example of WHP Activity in Britain

Department of Health	– launched 'Look After Your Heart' campaign 1987 – strategy to raise public awareness on heart disease and its prevention – employers encouraged to participate in scheme using LAYH Charter – link with HSE in 'Saving Lives: Our Healthier Nation' workplace initiatives – back injury prevention; healthy living centres
National Health Service	– contributes to 'Health at Work' initiatives – designated health promotion specialist
Health and Safety Executive	– mobilising legislation – work with government policy initiatives – advice and consultancy
CBI and TUC	– support and encouragement to members – endorses health related initiatives of the Department of Health and Health Promotion Departments
The Health Agencies, e.g. Health Promotion Wales/ Health Education Board Scotland/Health Education Authority England	- develops strategies for workplace health activities, e.g. 'Corporate Health/Corporate Action' – interprets and advises in government policies – advice to companies – standard and tailored health promotion programmes – maintains database relating to health development activity

Most occupational health professionals are from single discipline backgrounds and may be unfamiliar with the multi-disciplinary, participatory approach that health promotion demands and which could challenge current professional practice.

Springett and Dugdill 1995

Springett and Dugdill emphasised that health promotion has focussed largely on health assessment, screening and the control of hazards that threaten health.

This process was further emphasised in the *Health of the Nation* policy which stayed with traditional models of disease prevention and individual behaviour change.

WHP being ... Concerned with educating people about the reasons for ill health and helping them to adopt healthier lifestyles. Health promotion activity in the workplace is more than about occupational health; it is concerned with using opportunities that this setting provides to promote healthy lifestyles, behaviour and attitudes in everyday life outside of work. The workplace offers the potential to reach 22 million employees currently in work.

HoN Taskforce 1993

The HEA's (1997) perspective emphasises the issue of control and taking control over health.

The phrase 'workplace health promotion' covers those activities designed to improve health and reduce risk factors for employees. Health promotion emphasises gaining control over personal well being and encouraging an environment that fosters that control. Applied to the workplace, this means that healthy practices should be encouraged among individuals through education, but also that attention must be paid to developing and maintaining working conditions conducive to the well being of the workforce as a whole. Employers also have legal responsibility to protect employees both as individuals and as part of the workforce.

HEA 1997, p. 6

Issues and limitations

The approach is useful from an individual standpoint as recipients can benefit from the personal attention to their health needs and maintain some privacy. However, personal motivation is required and there is sole reliance on the individual for accounting for their health problems (victim blaming). Those involved with exercise or diet regimes with other colleagues may experience peer pressure.

This approach does not tackle broader issues in the work environment, i.e. conditions, poor policies, and oppressive working practices.

Multi-level approach

This approach focuses on the organisation as encompassing many facets which impinge upon the individual. It looks at the way in which the individual negotiates their work environment and identifies a problem solving approach to health issues. This largely includes mobilising existing resources such as occupational health services, personnel policy, work design issues and adherence to national legislation to maintain health at work.

Issues and limitations

The approach encourages complacency and the ethos of health improvement is lost in a disintegrated approach to health improvement. Attention to health improvement is largely mobilised when a problem is identified by individuals or through accident. There is little if any protection. The communication loop is not closed as issues become lost or dealt with by those with designated responsibility on a statutory basis to protect the workforce, further confining the health promotion–health improvement and development ethos. There is limited benefit to the organisation and the workforce as a whole.

Organisational approach

A popular approach with its origins in the Nordic countries. It is heavily reliant on initial analysis of health-related problems in the workplace. It encourages employee participation initiatives whereby negotiation and collaboration are necessary. Programmes are tailored and developed in accordance with perceived need. Competing requirements between the physical environment and the psychosocial components of the workplace and the individual employee are acknowledged. The approach is largely concerned with implementing changes in the workplace of both a structural and legislative nature, in order to create a more health promoting environment. The approach is intended to emphasise collaboration.

Issues and limitations

There is considerable attention to the health needs of the workforce as they are involved at all stages through to implementation and execution of strategies. The approach does, however, require a motivated workforce where a culture of health promotion is openly fostered.

Democratico-participatory approach

The essence of this approach is that it acknowledges the consideration of political goals. The first developed by Gardell encourages a process of decision making and forms of organisation to improve worker health.

The second, by Conrad, encourages social policy issues reflecting upon health inequalities crossing the work and home divide.

The first approach, developed by Gardell and Svensson in the 1970s in Stockholm, involves the development of a combined interdependent and mutually reinforcing ethos at a number of levels within the organisation. It emphasises workers' influence in the decision-making process in many aspects of working life. The approach instils political development and awareness of workers and comprises three elements:

1   *Autonomous groups* – the workforce are organised into groups depending on their specific range of expertise and are involved in jointly organising and planning their own work. Each member and their contribution is treated with equal value.
2   *Codetermination* – collective decision making occurs amongst managers and workers/workers' representatives in relation to personnel policy, work environment, production planning, company budget, technological development and recruitment.
3   *Individual self-determination* – each worker is responsible for organising the process of their own work including interchange and administration within departments.

The approach encouraged psychosocial health improvement largely through workers having more control and greater autonomy in the work undertaken and performed. Work was more flexible and absenteeism was known to decline sharply (Johnson and Johansson 1991).

Conrad identifies with the original notion of WHP in terms of definition, but later in developing his ideas refers to a structural emphasis because the notion of concentration on the individual alone has been found to be inadequate.

Conrad (1988) presents a slightly different perspective of WHP to Feilding. He refers to:

... A combination of educational, organisational and environmental activities designed to support behaviour conducive to the health of employees and their families. In effect ... [It] consists of health education, screening and/or intervention designed to change employee behaviour in a healthward direction and reduce the associated risks. It differs from the traditional occupational health mission in that wellness programs are interested in general health promotion among employees rather than focussing on health protection, i.e. preventing occupational diseases or insuring safe working conditions.

Conrad 1988, p. 485

The focus for Conrad relates to employees and their families. It is social in terms of approach and aims in the sense that it is assumed that whatever employees learn/receive concerning health issues at work, it will be cascaded down to the people they share their lives with outside the workplace. It is in essence bringing health to the community. For Conrad

The lifestyle risk factor approach to worksite health promotion has some pitfalls. For example, social scientists and health educators have very limited knowledge about how to change people's (healthy and unhealthy) habits. Education is helpful, but not sufficient. Most people are aware of the health risks of smoking or not wearing seat belts, yet roughly 30 per cent of Americans smoke and, when not required by law, 80 per cent don't regularly use seatbelts.

Conrad 1988, p. 487

Conrad undermines the view that individual risk and responsibility are solely and rarely the domain of the individual. He states that this merely reduces all health problems that emerge from work rest with the individual, so blaming the victim for their illness. He also states that practical health programmes which adhere to lifestyle behaviour change, e.g. healthy diet, exercise regimes are largely preaching to the converted and therefore resources provided by managers are not being channelled in the right direction. They ignore issues like social deprivation and social class, and have not been attractive to blue collar workers. Attention is shifted, it is claimed by health promoters, which can mask and ignore the health effects of working conditions. It is those situations and the work environment. The structural issues that require attention combined with programmes which target and reduce discrimination, social deprivation and isolation in the workplace.

There is now a general acceptance in the field of workplace health promotion that the mere provision of exercise and canteen facilities will not enhance behavioural and organisational change. The belief that defining workplace health promotion is difficult goes hand in hand with achievement; it is difficult because organisations are so geared towards accident prevention and are preoccupied with disease prevention. Much emphasis is placed on the individual to change their behaviour rather than to change the organisation's culture.

Specific worker's needs are not considered within the context of their work or issues of deprivation. How does one encourage those in manufacturing, shop workers and factory workers to think about, communicate and embrace health issues? Also those lower down the hierarchy of workplaces – what are they considering in terms of health?

Applications to British context

Not sure that health promotion on a corporate level in the British context is likely to dilute occupational health/health and safety because:

1   models of occupational health embrace an interest in health promotion, but may not be taking a health promotion approach in practice when other priorities are imminent;
2   the strong tradition in the UK of health and safety legislation and consciousness is more developed than health promotion. If anything, health promoters have worked hard to gain a foothold within organisations and to make known their approach and value as distinct from traditional methods;
3   health promotion is not taken to any fully developed way in the UK is it is still in the process of development. Each authority has its own interpretation. The issue of lifestyle and behaviour change is becoming a dated concept.

Like Conrad, a structuralist approach is emphasised by Health Promotion Wales (1995) but they develop this notion further, advocating wellness through permeating policy and process in organisations.

Health promotion in the workplace involves making a commitment to a healthier workforce by providing information and having policies and practices which assist employees to make healthy choices. It also involves recognising the impact that organisations can have on individuals.

... a healthy organisation successfully balances corporate and individual goals. It actively promotes health, has an open and flexible culture, seeks to reduce stress, recognises merit and rewards achievement.

Dwr Cymru, HPW, etc. 1995, p. 4

Health Promotion Wales' concept underlines the combined approach to health improvement. Tackling the structure in terms of policies, procedures and practices, and subsequent impact on the individual, will yield greater benefit.

Issues and limitations

Again this approach is reliant on worker motivation and a large amount of compliance to needs and expectations of the group as opposed to the individual or the organisation, although the structure ultimately is designed to improve flexibility at work and foster a more conducive working relationship that relieves boredom, alienation and stress. Achieving democracy for all in the workforce is a difficult process where issues of power, domination and control over advancement and resources are competing with external pressures from customers and family requirements. To date, the rate of success has been limited (Braverman 1974; Edwards 1979; Svensson 1984; Karlsson 1985).

Business planning approach

This approach was pioneered by Kizer in the US during the late 1980s. It is more popularly known as the SANE approach depicting specific elements of *Smoking and Alcohol policy development and Nutrition and Exercise issues*, although it is recognised that other elements are included. The plan is designed to stimulate thought about the needs of the company and its employees in an analytical way so there is an element of realism introduced into any health initiative. Looking at the company and the needs of industry immediately identifies problems, issues, external and internal competition.

The needs of the entire workforce in terms of health development and improvement are also ascertained through specially formulated corporate questionnaires. They range from specific health needs of the individual to the range of programmes available to the workforce, having sought specific guidance from health professionals external to the organisation. This detailed information is processed by the organisation to develop a corporate plan which takes account of broader company objectives. The strategic planning element builds in long and short term goals, as well as identifying priorities, training, and participatory funding elements. The management team are devolved to devise the timetable, set up and communicate elements of the programme, and encourage worker participation. They will also be involved in evaluating and monitoring the outcome of initiatives.

The evaluation of the programme looks at the economic aspects. A financial analysis is undertaken in terms of expenditure measured against sickness, absence of employees over a given period of time.

The evaluative element also includes a company audit in terms of effectiveness of the programme, the cycle of planning, support for the programme, and impact on employee health (Figure 2).

Similar programmes are now being used in Britain but their development is not so advanced.

Issues and limitations

Since health promotion is built into the corporate culture, the likelihood of success is greater. This is predominantly the case when there is managerial support for health promotion (Wynne and Clarkin 1992; Breuker 1998).

Specific elements can be built into the programme as and when the company feel it is necessary, so there is a large element of control. This may, on reflection, become a rather closed process as there is no guarantee that the company will keep up to date with the latest health improvements or policies which are nationally led. The company may benefit from assistance either from their local public health department, or may employ a health promotion specialist working jointly with the company and the health authority. This way, the company maintains contact with community and national health development and the health authority broker a relationship to maintain research, development and publication of advances in health improvement within companies. This, however, would require greater development as piloting such work is not readily apparent in the current literature.

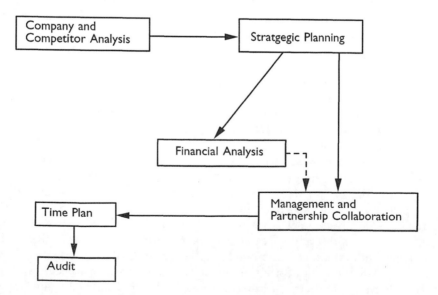

Figure 2 Adapted from Kizer's Business Plan for Health Promotion (1987).

Is there a need for health promotion at work?

During the financial year 1992/1993, there were 627.2 million days of certi-fied incapacity in Great Britain due to sickness and invalidity – 436.5 million for men and 190.7 million for women. These figures refer largely to periods of reported illness. Short spells of illness lasting fewer than 4 days would not generally be reported to the Department, therefore these figures underesti-mate the actual number of working days lost as a result of sickness. Sickness figures are also affected by the national economic situation, as those at risk of losing their jobs are less likely to take time off for genuine ill health than those who feel secure.

Increasing management attention to sickness absence also puts pressure on people to remain at work, return to work or retire from work when they have health conditions that would otherwise have been tolerated.

In both men and women, diseases of the musculo-skeletal system are the commonest cause of absence. While in men diseases of the circulatory system is the second commonest cause, for women it is mental disorders. The single greatest cause of disease for which statistics are available is coronary heart disease, at 58.4 million days lost for men and 7.6 million for women (Bunt 1993; Department of Employment 1993; Office of National Statistics 1996).

In a typical year in Britain, it is estimated that 80 million days are lost annually as a result of stress-related illness, 35 million days for coronary heart disease and 3.6 million days for back pain, compared with the loss of only 761,000 working days because of strikes in 1991 (CSO 1995). DSS statistics for 1993/1994 show that back pain accounted for 106 million days of certified incapacity for work (HSE 1995).

A detailed study of sickness absence in civil servants (CSO 1995) concluded that recognised risk factors seem to explain only a third of the large differences in sickness absence between the higher and lower grades of civil servants, with the lower grades taking from three to six times more sickness absence.

The recognised risk factors were smoking and frequent consumption of alcohol, work characteristics (that is, the level of control they felt they had, the amount of variety and how well their skills were used, the pace of work and the level of support they had at work), low levels of job satisfaction and adverse social circumstances outside work (financial difficulties and negative support).

There is also increasing emphasis on the psychosocial health problems at the workplace. A UNISON Report (1997) underlined the increasing rise of harassment and bullying in the workplace as a result of their race, creed or sex. They found that

- 1 in 7 of its members were being bullied;
- 14 per cent of unison members are being bullied in any 6 month period (in a third of these cases, bullying had gone on for at least 3 years);

- 92 per cent of respondents think bullying is caused by overwork (University of Staffordshire and IRS 1997).

RONIN Research Services in 1997 surveyed a number of companies in Britain, and of 1043 people they contacted, over half had received flame mails. These were usually sent by managers. Men were regarded as the main perpetrators and there were more women on the receiving end of offensive mail. This led to stress, loss of confidence, loss of productivity and an avoidance of face to face communication with colleagues (IRS 1997).

Evaluation of WHP programmes

Workplace health promotion activity has suffered in the past because of limited evaluation of the effectiveness of activities. Indeed, it has been recognised by some experts that if programme costs cannot be justified through evaluation results, then cancellation of workplace health promotion programmes during times of economic recession is more likely to occur (Eddy et al. 1989).

To date, health promotion practice in the workplace has lacked rigour, with many activities taking place in isolation. Rarely is such activity part of a co-ordinated strategy with an integrated approach to problem analysis, programme planning, implementation and evaluation procedures (Springett and Dugdill 1995).

Those studies which have been evaluated, have for the most part been concerned with reduced absenteeism and staff turnover. Betera's study looked at absenteeism amongst full time employees in a large multi-location, diversified industrial population. Blue collar employees participating in a comprehensive health promotion intervention experienced 14 per cent decline in absenteeism over a 2 year period, compared with a 5.8 per cent decline showed by a control group (Betera 1990).

The US Department of Health and Human Services (1993) conducted a survey of employers to ascertain findings regarding workplace health promotion activity. Workplaces of 50 or more employees, i.e. 1,507 workplaces, found that in terms of evaluation, 49 per cent of workplaces analyse health care costs prior to implementation of activity, 27 per cent conduct needs assessment.

Only 28 per cent examine death and disability reports. Only 31 per cent kept records of health promotion activities and only 12 per cent conduct formal evaluation.

Frameworks for evaluation of workplace health activity are being developed in Britain. The ones currently reported draw largely on work undertaken in the US, Sweden, the Netherlands and Canada (Israel et al. 1989; Hugentobler et al. 1992; Wynne and Clarkin 1992; Springett and Dugdill 1995). It has yet to be formally tested in the UK, but undoubtedly will act as a catalyst for further health related activity in the workplace, and hopefully encourage a broadened concept of workplace health promotion.

Implementation and evaluation of programmes is an area of particular difficulty, not merely because of a lack of appropriate framework to suit specific climates, but also because managers tend to prefer singular initiatives that boost the image of the organisation rather than long term considerations (Wilkinson 1997).

WHP in Europe

The EU Framework Directive on Health and Safety compels the employer to recognise stress factors and to correct them. This framework states, amongst other things, that the employer has

> a duty to ensure the safety and health of workers in every aspect related to the work, following general principles of prevention: avoiding risks, evaluating the risks which cannot be avoided, combating the risk at source, adapting the work to the individual, especially as regards the design of workplaces, the choice of work equipment and the choice of working and production methods, with a view in particular to alleviating monotonous work and work at a predetermined work rate and to reducing their effect on health.
>
> EU Framework Directive on Health and Safety pp. 26–27

Stress is a problem for the worker and the organisation. It leads to sickness, absence and disability; underlines a poor working climate. Increasing flexibilisation of the workforce, new technologies, increasing mental effort and contributory factors. It is a legal obligation in some EU countries to deal with stress. Increasing globalisation means a necessity to improve productivity and quality at work (Kompier and Levi 1994).

What constitutes a health promotion programme in the workplace?

There are a series of activities that may constitute a health promotion programme, however, they are generally considered to be so if the following criteria are met:

1 the activities are designed to improve or maintain health of employees, dependents and retirees;
2 participation is voluntary;
3 programmes involve activities in addition to the provision of educational materials;

4   programmes address one or more factors reasonably demonstrated to alter personal health risk; and
5   programmes are offered on a periodic or continuing basis. (Feilding 1991, in Green and Baker).

Within the last decade a series of activities across Europe have stimulated interest in workplace health, predominantly through the goodwill of individual organisations and through European Public Health Policy. A proposal submitted to the European Parliament and Council was accepted in 1996. The proviso is that such programmes must demonstrate importance to the Community as a whole which extends beyond national priorities and policies. This too has been realised in the workplace through the formulation of a Network.

Much of the developments relating to workplace health and health and safety improvements in recent years across the European Union has been influenced by public health policy outlined by the European Commission. Article 129 of the Treaty on European Union states that:

1   The community shall contribute towards a high level of human health protection by encouraging co-operation between the member states and if necessary lending support to their action. Community action shall be directed towards the prevention of diseases, in particular the major health scourges, including drug dependence by promoting research into their causes and their transmission as well as health information and education.

    Health protection requirements shall form a constituent part of the Community's other policies.

2   Member states shall, in liaison with the Commission, co-ordinate among themselves their policies and programmes in the areas referred to in paragraph 1: The Commission may, in close contact with the member states take any useful initiative to promote such co-ordination.
3   The Community and the Member States shall foster co-operation with third countries and the competent international organisations in the sphere of public health.
4   In order to contribute to the achievement of the objectives referred to in the Article, the Council: acting in accordance with the procedure referred to in Article 189b after consulting the Economic and Social Committee and the Committee of the Regions, shall adopt incentive measures, excluding any harmonisation of the laws and regulations of the member states (European Commission 1997).

The European Commission has developed proposals to action a health promotion programme, and having being taken through the European Parliament and Commission, was adopted on 16th February 1996.

A 5 year programme costing ECU 35 million was established. Work place health promotion was a small part of this and the basic principles underpinning the *main strategy* are as follows:

Health promotion at work is intended to help healthier practices and behaviour at work to become easier and more rewarding for all concerned.1. A corporate culture and philosophy which accords the workforce's health the same priority as the enterprise's economic goals creates a good atmosphere for a comprehensive policy to promote health within the enterprise. In particular, this involves guidelines for co-operative and participative methods of management practice which accords high priority to the well being of workers.2. A health and safety policy which places the emphasis on prevention and is refined to produce forward looking, health conscious job design provides a good platform for overall health promotion at work.3. Personnel deployment and development strategies enable the potential offered by these technical and organisational aspects of work to be exploited to the full.4. The enterprise's social policy encourages co-operation amongst workers, involvement in health insurance schemes on all matters of health protection; expert advice for people suffering from psychosocial stress and addiction problems; widening the range of facilities of work for exercise and relaxation.5. Arrangements in working hours should be conducive to family and work demands. The reduction of stress is of importance when considering the differing roles of men and women. Humane planning of shifts and arrangements to reintroduce normal working hours for shift workers and especially night workers.6. Environment and health conscious production methods, products and services are part of the comprehensive health policy of such enterprises which seek to enhance their image locally and amongst customers and consumers.7. Health conscious organisations are encouraged to take an active role in municipal and regional health promotion, providing, for example, advice, practical help with premises or tools or sponsorship for municipal social and sports facilities.
Adapted from 'Public Health in Europe' European Commission 1997

As a result of developments in public health policy, members of the European Network for Workplace Health Promotion at a network meeting held in November 1997, founded the *Luxembourg Declaration on Workplace Health Promotion in the European Union*. It identified the broad ethos of the movement:

Workplace Health Promotion (WHP) is the combined efforts of employers, employees and society to improve the health and well being of people at work. This can be achieved through a combination of:
– improving the work organisation and the working environment
– promoting active participation
– encouraging personal development

The recent activity in this field emanates from two factors. Firstly, the Framework Directive on Safety and Health (Council Directive 89/391/EC) which provided a platform to alter traditional occupational health practice and legislation. Secondly, advancing the view that the workplace be regarded as a public health setting. These ideas are not new, however, the *Network* has been involved in raising the profile of health improvement activity in the work environment across Europe in a much more concerted and collaborative way than their colleagues in the US for example. The *Network* also intend to identify and disseminate examples of good practice.

The strategy under the *Declaration* aims, within a health promoting framework, to prevent ill health at work which includes accidents, occupational diseases and stress. More specifically, a holistic approach is taken in terms of development, planning and implementation of activity. Firstly, in adopting management principles and methods which involves investing in employees' knowledge and skills. Secondly, fostering a culture where there is leadership which combines participation, and encourages motivation and responsibility amongst employees. Thirdly, establishing work organisation principles which provide the workforce with an appropriate balance between job demands, control over their work, provision of social support and development of skills. Finally, making use of established services within the workplace to channel health promotion and occupational health issues.

The World Health Organization's contribution to WHP

The WHO's initial interest in workplace health improvement was announced in the 40th World Health Assembly in 1987 which requested the Director General in resolution WHA 40.28 to

pay attention to workers' health programmes and to develop guidelines on health promotion in the workplace ... employers and managers should recognize that health promotion in the workplace is in the interest of both employers and workers, and should take the initiative in collaborating with workers and workers' representatives to implement health promotion programmes.

WHO 1988, p. 2

Despite this pronouncement in the late 1980s, it is only over a decade later that guidance has been provided by the WHO which dovetails with other WHP strategies (Wilkinson 1999). The reasons for under development are apparent and have already been covered elsewhere in this book, but they largely relate to fragmentation, difference in the needs of different enterprises, lack of political will in some instances and the dominance of occupational medicine (Wynne 1993).

The WHO now considers the workplace as a priority setting for health promotion and improvement in the twenty-first century.

So why now?

As indicated in Chapter 4, the nature of work is changing. The workforce of the world today exceeds 2.7 billion people. Some 80 per cent are in countries that are still developing (WHO 1995). Despite increasing industrialisation, many of these workers will be found in subsistence agriculture. Economic development may contribute to improved health; however, unplanned and poorly controlled industrialisation increases health risks. Health impact assessment will be required to reposition industries where pollution does not affect the general health of population of communities and the transfer of unsafe products and practices to other countries (WHO 1997). New strategies will be required to increase access to WHP in developing countries among both agricultural and industrial workforce.

There is also an increasingly ageing workforce, and a progressive number of women entering the workplace. Knowledge and literacy is also improving which means more people can contribute to new forms of work. Technological innovations alter patterns of working and availability of employment. This means increasing numbers of small and medium sized enterprises, increasing part time work, informal working, and self employment. These issues and environments bring with them their own health issues and pressures which are likely to impact on the workforce, planning and management.

Technological innovation also brings with it the issue of adaptability and unemployment. There is currently an estimated job shortage of 1.3 billion around the world. Unemployment has its specific psychosocial and health problems which emanate from insecurity and instability.

WHO's health promoting ethos

The WHO take their lead on workplace health development and improvement by building on the philosophies of the Ottawa Charter and specific activity already undertaken within the workplace that improves the health needs and conditions of workers. It includes a number of dynamic issues.

WHO WHP Ethos
- Creating health-promoting policies
  - This occurs within regional, national, and other priorities, e.g. European Union Framework Directive; Well Works Project (USA).
  - Internal organisation policies relating to alcohol misuse, smoking, HIV/AIDS and safety.
- Creating supportive environments.
  - Commitment and leadership inside the work environment and from governments
  - Action to promote a safe and healthy working environment.
  - Access to safe drinking water and basic sanitation.
  - Appropriate work design and organisation.
- Strengthening workplace action
  - Encouraging worker participation in planning and implementing WHP programmes.
  - Recognition of non-occupational factors that impact on the health and well being of others, e.g. literacy, the family, violence.
- Developing personal skills
  - For protection against the effects of stress, substance abuse and the promotion of healthy dietary intake and exercise.
  - Provision of training to enable successful implementation of WHP programmes.
- Strengthening health services
  - Working in partnership with health services to increase access to primary care, occupational health services, service users.

Adapted from 'The Health-Promoting Workplace:
Making It Happen' (WHO 1998)

As you can see from this chapter, workplace health promotion is still developing and no doubt in time the approaches will expand and stabilise. In the interim period, it is hoped that research will continue into all phenomena of workplace health improvement.

References

Adams A. (1992) *Bullying at Work*. London: Virago Press.

Adams J.S. (1965) Injustice in social exchange. In L. Berkowitz (editor), *Advances in Experimental Social Psychology*. New York: Academic Press.

Aglietta M. (1976) *A Theory of Capitalist Regulation: The US Experience* (Translated by David Ferbach). London: NLB.

Agricola (1556) *De Re Metallica*.

Akerstedt T. (1979) Altered sleep / wake patterns and circadian rhythms. Laboratory and field studies of sympathoadrenomedullary and related variables. *Acta Physiologica Scandinavia* Supplement 469.

Allende S. (1939) *La Realidad Medico – Social Chileno*. Ministerio de Salubidad, Prevision y Asistencia Social, Santiago (English Translation).

Arendt H. (1958a) *The Human Condition*. Chicago, IL: Chicago University Press.

Arendt H. (1958b) *The Origins of Totalitarianism*. New York: Viking Press.

Argyris C. (1951) *Personality and Organisation*. New York: Harper and Row.

Argyris C. (1964) *Integrating the Individual and the Organisation*. New York: Wiley.

Aronowitz S. (1974) *False Promises: The Shaping of American Working Class Consciousness*. New York: McGraw–Hill.

Arthur R.J. and Grunderson E.K. (1965) Promotion and mental illness in the Navy. *Journal of Occupational Medicine* 7, 452–456.

Atkinson J. and Meager N. (1986) *Changing Working Patterns: How Companies Achieve Flexibility to Meet New Needs*. London: NEDO.

Averill J.R. (1973) Personal control over aversive stimuli and its relationship to stress. *Psychology Bulletin* 80, 286–303.

Bainton C.R. and Peterson D.R. (1963) Deaths from coronary heart disease in persons fifty years of age and younger: a community-wide study. *New England Journal of Medicine* 268, 569–574.

Baker E., Israel B.A. and Schurman S. (1996) The integrated model: implications for worksite health promotion and occupational health and safety. *Health Education Quarterly* 23 (2), 175–190.

Barratt E.S. (1990) Human resource management: organisational culture. *Management Update* 2 (1), 21–32.

Battiscombe G. (1974) *Shaftesbury: A Biography of the Seventh Earl 1801–1885*. London: Constable.

Beckhard R. (1969) *Organisation Development: Strategies and Models.* Reading, MA: Addison-Wesley.

Bendelow G. and Williams S.J. (1998) *Emotions in Social Life: Critical Themes and Contemporary Issues.* London: Routledge.

Berkson D. (1960) Socioeconomic correlates of atherosclerotic and hypertensive heart disease in culture, society and health. *Annals of New York Academy of Science* 84, 835–850.

Betera R.I. (1990) Planning and implementing health promotion in the workplace: a case study of the Du Pont company experience. *Health Education Quarterly* 17 (3), 307–327.

Beynon H. (1973) *Working for Ford.* Harmondsworth: Penguin.

Black D., Morris J.N. and Townsend P. (1980) *The Black Report.* London: HMSO.

Blauner R. (1964) *Alienation and Freedom.* Chicago, IL: Chicago University Press.

Bosch G. (1995) *Social Europe: Flexibility and Work Organisation.* Supplement 1: 95, European Commission.

Boumans N.P.G. and Landeweerd J.A. (1993) Leadership in the nursing unit: relationships with nurses' well being. *Journal of Advanced Nursing* 18, 767–775.

Bowey A. (1976) *The Sociology of Organisations.* London: Hodder and Stoughton.

Bowles S. and Gintis H. (1976) *Schooling in Capitalist America: Educational Reform and the Contradictions of Economic Life.* New York: Basic Books.

Bradley G. (1983) Effects of computerisation on work environment and health. *Occupational Health Nursing* 31 (11), 35–39.

Braverman H. (1974) *Labour and Monopoly Capital: The Degradation of Work in the Twentieth Century.* New York: Monthly Review Press.

Breslow L. and Buell P. (1960) Mortality from coronary heart disease and physical activity of work in California. *Journal of Chronic Disease* 11, 615–626.

Breslow L. and Feilding J. (1983) Health promotion programs, sponsored by California employers. *American Journal of Public Health* 73, 538–542.

Breslow L., Fielding J., Herrmann A.A. and Wilbur C.S. (1990) Worksite health promotion: its evaluation and the Johnson and Johnson experience. *Preventive Medicine* 19, 13–21.

Brown I. (1985) Ergonomics and technological change. *Ergonomics* 28 (9), 1301–1309.

Buck V. (1972) *Working Under Pressure.* London: Staples.

Bulmer M. (1975) *Working Class Images of Society.* London: Routledge and Kegan Paul.

Burawoy M. (1979) *Manufacturing Consent: Changes in the Labour Process Under Monopoly Capitalism.* Chicago, IL: Chicago University Press.

Burns T. and Stalker G. (1961) *The Management of Innovation.* London: Tavistock Publications.

Burrell G. (1988) Modernism, post modernism and organisational analysis 2: the contribution of Michel Foucault. *Organisation Studies* 9 (2), 221–235.

Caplan R. (1975) Job *Demands and Worker Health.* Washington, DC: National Institute of Occupational Health and Safety (NIOSH).

Caplan R.P. (1994) Stress, anxiety and depression in hospital consultants, general practitioners and senior health service managers. *British Medical Journal* 309, 1261–1263.

Cassell J. (1974) The use of medical records: opportunities for epidemiological studies. *Journal of Occupational Medicine* 5, 185–190.

Caudhill W. (1958) *The Psychiatric Hospital as a Small Society.* Cambridge, MA: Harvard University Press.

Chambers R. and Belcher J. (1992) Work patterns of general practitioners before and after the introduction of the 1990 contract. *British Journal of General Practice* 43 (375), 410–412.

Child J. (1972) Organisational structure, environment and performance. *Sociology* 6 (1), 1–22.

Cleland L.G. (1987) RSI: a model of social iatrogenesis. *Medical Journal of Australia* 147, 236–239.

Clutterbuck R.C. (1980) Industrial ill health in the United Kingdom. *International Journal of Health Services* 10 (1), 149–161.

Coburn D. (1978) Work and general psychological and physical well being. *International Journal of Health Services* 8, 415–435.

Coburn D. (1979) Job alienation and well being. *International Journal of Health Services* 9, 41–59.

Cohen B.H. (1980) Chronic obstructive pulmonary disease: a challenge in genetic epidemiology. *American Journal of Epidemiology* 112, 274–288.

Cohen D. (1994) Health promotion and cost effectiveness. *Health Promotion International* 9 (4), 281–287.

COMA (1983) *Diet and Cardiovascular Disease.* Report on Health and Social Subjects, No. 28. London: HMSO.

Conrad P. (1987) Wellness in the workplace: potentials and pitfalls of worksite health promotion. *Milbank Quarterly* 65, 255–275.

Conrad P. (1988) Worksite health promotion. The social context. *Social Science and Medicine* 26 (5), 485–489.

Conrad R. (1960) Letter sorting machines – paced, "lagged" or unpaced? *Ergonomics* 3, 149–157.

Cooper C.L. (1973) *Group Training for Individual and Organisational Development.* Basel, Switzerland: Karger.

Cooper C.L. and Williams S. (1994) *Creating Health Work Organisations.* Chichester: Wiley.

Cooper R. (1989) Modernism, post modernism and organisational analysis 3: the contribution of Jacques Derrida. *Organisation Studies* 110 (4), 479–502.

Cooper R. and Burrell G. (1988) Modernism, postmodernism and organisational analysis. *Organisation Studies* 9 (1), 91–112.

Coren A. (1980) When work is soulless, life stifles and dies. In M. Dixon and I. Bodenheimer (editors), *Health Care in Crisis.* San Francisco, CA: Synthesis.

Cotgrove S. (1972) Alienation and automation. *British Journal of Sociology* December.

Dalton M. (1959) *Men Who Manage.* New York: Wiley.

Davidson R. (1970) *Peril on the Job: A Study of Hazards in the Chemical Industries.* Washington, DC: Public Affairs Press.

Dawson S. (1988) *Safety At Work: The Limits of Self Regulation.* Cambridge, MA: Cambridge University Press.

De Man H. (1929) *Joy in Work* (translated by E. Paul and C. Paul). London: George Allen and Unwin.

Deal T.E. and Kennedy A.A. (1982) *Corporate Cultures: The Rites and Rituals of Corporate Life*. Reading, MA: Addison-Wesley.

Denison D.R. (1984) Bringing corporate culture to the bottom line. *Organisational Dynamics* 13 (2), 5–22.

Department of Health (1998a) *Saving Lives: Our Healthier Nation*. London: Stationery Office.

Department of Health (1998b) *The New NHS: Modern and Dependable*. London: Stationery Office.

Derrida J. (1973) *Speech and Phenomena*. Evanston: North Western University Press.

Derrida J. (1978) *Writing and Difference*. London: Tavistock Publications.

Drucker P.F. (1981) The coming rediscovery of scientific management. In P.F. Drucker (editor), *The Conference Board Record*, Vol. XIII, June 1976. *Towards the Next Economics and Other Essays*. Heinemann, pp. 23–27.

Dubin R. (1956) Industrial workers worlds: a study of the central life interests of industrial workers. *Social Problems* 3.

Durkheim E. (1947) *The Division of Labour* (originally published in 1893). New York: Free Press.

Durkheim E. (1952) *Suicide, A Study in Sociology* (originally published in 1897). London: Glencoe.

Eddy J.M., Gold R.S. and Zimmerli W.H. (1989) Evaluation of worksite health enhancement programmes. *Health Values: Achieving High Levels of Wellness* 13 (1), 3, 9.

Emerson H. (1913) *The Twelve Principles of Efficiency*. New York: Engineering Magazine Company.

Engels F. (1844) *The Condition of the Working Class in England* (revised version 1987). London: Penguin.

Engels F. (1845) *The Conditions of the Working Class in England*. London: Penguin.

Engels F. (1973) *Condition of the Working Class in England*. London: Penguin.

European Commission (1998) *New Forms of Work Organisation: Case Studies*. Final Report, June, Luxembourg.

Eyer J. (1975) Hypertension as a disease of modern society. *International Journal of Health Services* 5 (4), 539–558.

Eyer J. (1977) Prosperity as a cause of death. *International Journal of Health Services* 7 (1), 125–150.

Eyer J. (1984) Capitalism, health and illness. In J.B. McKinlay (editor), *Illness in the Political Economy of Health Care*. London: Tavistock Publications.

Eyer J. and Karasek J. (1979) Job decision latitude, job demands and cardiovascular disease: a prospective study of Swedish men. *American Journal of Public Health* 70, 694–705.

Eyer J. and Karasek J. (1984) Co-worker and supervisor support as moderators of associations between task and characteristics and mental strain. *Journal of Occupational Behaviour* 3, 147–160.

Eyer J. and Sterling P. (1977) Stress related mortality and social organisation. *Review of Radical Political Economics* 9 (1), 1–44.

Fairburn J. and McGettigan J. (1994) Development of an occupational health management model part 1. *Occupational Health Journal* 46 (4), 120–123.

Fayol H. (1918) *General and Industrial Management*. London: Pitman.

Feildstein A., Valanis B., Vollmer W., Stevens N. and Overton C. (1993) The back injury prevention project pilot study: assessing the effectiveness of back attack and injury prevention programs among nurses, aides and orderlies. *Journal of Occupational Medicine* 35, 114–120.

Feinleib M. and Kannel W. (1980) The relationship of psychosocial factors to coronary heart disease in the Framingham Study. *American Journal of Epidemiology* 111 (1), 37–58.

Ferguson D.A. (1987) RSI: putting the epidemic to rest. *Medical Journal of Australia* 47, 213–214.

Fielding J. (1984) *Corporate Health Management*. Reading, MA: Addison-Wesley.

Fielding J. (1991) Occupational health physicians and prevention. *Journal of Occupational Medicine* 33 (3), 314–326.

Firth-Cozens J. (1987) Emotional distress in junior house officers. *British Medical Journal* 295, 533–536.

Firth-Cozens J. (1995) *Stress in Doctors; a Longitudinal Study*. University of Leeds.

Fischer S. (1984) *Stress and The Perception of Control*. Hillsdale, NJ: Lawrence Erlbaum.

Fortes M. (1962) Ritual and office in tribal society. In M. Gluckman (editor), *Essays on the Ritual of Social Relations*. Manchester, UK: University of Manchester Press, pp. 53–89.

Foucault M. (1973) *The Birth of the Clinic*. London: Tavistock Publications.

Foucault M. (1980) *Power/Knowledge*. Brighton, UK: Harvester.

Frampton K. (1979) The status of man and the status of his objects: a reading of the human condition. In M.A. Hill (editor), *Hannah Arendt: The Recovery of the Public World*. New York: St. Martins Press.

Francis M.E. and Pennebaker J.W. (1992) Putting stress into words: the impact of writing on psychological, absentee and self reported emotional well being measures. *American Journal of Health Promotion* 6 (4), 280–287.

Frankenhauser M. (1986) Psychobiological framework for research on human stress and coping. In M.H. Appleby and R. Trumball (editors), *Dynamics of Stress*. New York: Plenum, pp. 101–116.

Frankenhauser M. (1988) To err is human: nuclear war by mistake? In A. Gromyko and M. Hellman (editors), *Breakthrough: Emerging New Thinking*. New York: Walker, pp. 53–60.

Frankenhauser M. (1991) *A Biopsychosocial Approach to Work Life Issues*. New York: Baywood Publishing Co.

Frankenhauser M. and Gardell B. (1976) Overload and underload in working life: outline of a multidisciplinary approach. *Journal of Human Stress* 2 (3), 35–45.

Freidmann F.A. and Havighurst R.J. (1954) *The Meaning of Work in Retirement*. Chicago, IL: Chicago University Press.

French J.R.P. and Caplan R. (1970) Psychosocial factors in coronary heart disease. *Industrial Medicine* 39, 383–397.

French J.R.P. and Caplan R. (1972) Organisational stress and individual strain. In A. Marrow (editor), *The Failure of Success*. New York: AMACOM, pp. 30–66.

French J.R.P. and Caplan R.D. (1973) Organisational stress and individual strain. In A.J. Marrow (editor), *The Failure of Success*, second edition. New York: AMACOM.

French J.R.P., Tupper C.J. and Mueller E.I. (1965) *Workload of University Professors*. Ann Arbor, MI: University of Michigan Press.

Friedlander F. (1967) Importance of work versus non-work during socially and occupationally stratified groups. *Journal of Applied Psychology* 50.

Friedman A.L. (1977) *Industry and Labour: Class Struggle at Work and Monopoly Capitalism*. New York: MacMillan.

Friend B. (1990) Working at health. *Nursing Times* 86, 21.

Frith H. and Kitzinger C. (1998) Emotion work as a participant resource: a feminist analysis of young women's talk-in-interaction. *Sociology* 32 (2), 299–320.

Gallie D. (1978) *In Search of the New Working Class: Automation and Social Integration in the Capitalist Enterprise*. Cambridge, MA: Cambridge University Press.

Gardell B. (1966) Plant relocation, personnel planning, and employee reaction. *Personnel Administration* 29 (5), 41–44.

Gardell B. (1971) Technology, alienation and mental health in the modern industrial environment. In L. Levi (editor), *Society, Stress and Disease*, Vol. 1. *The Psychosocial Environment and Psychosomatic Diseases*. London: Oxford University Press, pp. 148–180.

Gardell B. (1976a) *Job Content and the Quality of Life*. Stockholm: Uppsala University Press.

Gardell B. (1976b) Technology, alienation and mental health. Summary of a social psychological research programme on technology and the worker. *Acta Sociologica* 19, 83–94.

Gardell B. (1977a) Autonomy and participation at work. *Human Relations* 30, 515–533.

Gardell B. (1977b) Psychosocial and social problems of industrial work in affluent societies. *International Journal of Psychology* 12, 125–134.

Gardell B. (1980) Autonomy and participation at work. In I.D. Katz, R. Kahn and J.C. Adams (editors), *The Study of Organisations*. San Francisco, CA: Jossey-Bass.

Gardell B. (1982a) Scandinavian research on stress in working life. *International Journal of Health Services* 12 (1), 31–41.

Gardell B. (1982b) Worker participation and autonomy: a multilevel approach to democracy at the workplace. *International Journal of Health Services* 12 (4), 527–558.

Gardell B. (1987) *Work Organisation and Human Nature: A Review of Research on Man's Need to Control Technlogy*. Stockholm: Swedish Work Environment Fund.

Gardell B. and Gustafson R.A. (1979) *Assembly Line Health Care. A Research Project on the Organisation of Care and Work in Hospital*. Stockholm: University of Stockholm.

Gardell B. and Gustavsen B. (1980) Work environment research and social change. Current developments in Scandinavia. *Journal of Occupational Behaviour* 1, 3–17.

Gardell B. and Gustavsen B. (1982) Worker participation and autonomy: a multilevel approach to democracy at the workplace. *International Journal of Health Services* 12 (4), 527–558.

Gardell B. and Svensson L. (1981) *Codetermination and Autonomy: A Local Trade Union Strategy for Democracy at the Workplace*. Stockholm: Prism.

Gardner B.B. (1945) *Human Relations in Industry*. Chicago, IL: Richard D. Irwin.

Garfield J. (1978) *The Organisation of Work and The Risk of Coronary Disease*. Paper presented at the 106th Annual Meeting of the American Public Health Association, October 16th 1978, Los Angeles.

Garfield J. (1979) Social stress and medical ideology. In C.A. Garfield (editor), *Stress and Survival: The Emotional Realities of Life Threatening Illness*. St. Louis, MO: C.V. Mosby, pp. 33–44.

Garfield J. (1980) Alienated labour, stress and coronary disease. *International Journal of Health Services* 10 (4), 551–561.

Garfinkel H. (1956) Conditions of successful degradation ceremonies. *American Sociological Review* 61, 420–425.

Gephart R.J. (1978) Status degradation and organisational succession: an ethnomethodological approach. *Administrative Science Quarterly* 23rd December, 553–581.

Gerhardt U. (1989) *Ideas About Health and Illness*. Beverley Hills, CA: Sage.

Giddens A. (1988) *Capitalism and Modern Social Theory: An Analysis of Marx, Durkheim and Weber*. Cambridge, MA: Cambridge University Press.

Gillespie R. (1991) *Manufacturing Knowledge: A History of the Hawthorne Experiments*. Cambridge, MA: Cambridge University Press.

Ginsburg N. (1996) Social Europe – a new model of welfare? *European Dossier Series*, No. 44. University of North London.

Glasgow R.E., Terborg J.R., Hollis J.F., Sevenson H.H. and Boles S.M. (1995) Take heart: results from the initial phase of a worksite wellness program. *American Journal of Public Health* 86, 209–216.

Goldenhar L.M. and Schulte P.A. (1994) Intervention research in occupational health and safety. *Journal of Occupational Medicine* 36, 763–775.

Goldthorpe J.H. and Lockwood D. (1975) Sources of variation in working class images of society. In M. Bulmer (editor), *Working Class Images of Society*. London: Routledge and Kegan Paul.

Gorz A. (1965) Work and consumption. In P. Anderson and R. Blackburn (editors), *Towards Socialism*. London: Collins.

Gottlieb N. and McLeroy K.R. (1994) Social health. In M.P. O'Donnell (editor), *Health Promotion in the Workplace*. Albany, NY: Delmar.

Green G.M. and Baker F. (1991) *Work, Health and Productivity*. Oxford: Oxford University Press.

Grieco A. (1986) Sitting posture: an old problem and a new one. *Ergonomics* 29, 345–362.

Grint K. (1998) *The Sociology of Work*, second edition. Cambridge, MA: Polity Press.

Grossman R. and Scala K. (1993) Health promotion and organisational development–developing settings for health. In IFF (editors), *European Health Promotion Series*, No. 2. Vienna: WHO/Europe.

Gustavsen B. (1980) From satisfaction to collective action: trends in the development of research and reform in working life. *Economic Industrial Democracy* 1 (2), 147–170.

Gustavsen B. (1988) Workplace reform and democratic dialogue. *Economic Industrial Democracy* 6 (4), 456–480.

Gustavsen B. and Gardell B. (1980) Work environment research and social change: current developments in Scandinavia. *Journal of Occupational Behaviour* 1.

Gustavsen B. and Hunnius G. (1981) *New Patterns of Work Reform: The Case of Norway.* Oslo: Oslo University Press.

Hagberg M. (1987) *Occupational Shoulder and Neck Disorders.* Stockholm: The Swedish Work Environment Fund.

Hall E. (1991) *Gender, Work Control and Stress: A Theoretical Discussion and An Emprical Test.* New York: Baywood Publishing.

Handy C. (1985) *Understanding Organisations.* London: Penguin.

Harrison B. (1996) *Not Only The Dangerous Trades: Women's Work and Health In Britain, 1880–1914.* London: Taylor and Francis.

Harrison R. (1972) Understand your organisation's character. *Harvard Business Review* 50 (3), 119–128.

Haycox A. (1994) A methodology for estimating the costs and benefits of health promotion. *Health Promotion International* 9 (1), 5–11.

Haynes S. (1980) Women, work and coronary heart disease: prospective findings from the Framingham Heart Study (Part 3). *American Journal of Epidemiology* 111 (1), 37–58.

Health and Safety Executive (1976) *IFF Survey.* UK: HSE.

Health Canada (1992) *The Small Business Health Model–A Guide to Developing and Implementing Workplace Health System in Small Business.* Ottawa: Health Canada.

Health of the Nation Taskforce (1993) *The Health of the Nation Taskforce Report,* September 1993.

Henry J. (1963) *Culture Against Man.* New York: Random House.

Hersey P. and Blanchard K. (1988) *Management of Organisational Behaviour: Utilising Human Resources.* Englewood Cliffs, NJ: Prentice-Hall.

Herzberg F. (1966) *Work and the Nature of Man.* New York: Staples Press.

Herzberg F. (1968) *Work and the Nature of Man,* second edition. New York: Staples Press.

Hirst P. and Zeitlin J. (1991) Flexible specialisation versus post-fordism: theory, evidence and policy implication. *Economy and Society* 20 (1), 1–52.

Hochschild A.R. (1983) *The Managed Heart: Commercialisation of Human Feeling.* Berkeley, CA: University of California Press.

Hofstede G. (1991) *Cultures and Organisations: Software of the Mind.* London: McGraw–Hill.

Hoggett P. (1990) Modernisation, political straegy and the welfare state. *Studies In Decentralisation and Quasi-Markets,* No. 2. School for Advanced Urban Studies, University of Bristol.

Hugentobler M.K., Israel B.A., Shurman S.J. (1992) An action research approach to workplace health: integrating methods. *Health Education Quarterly* 19 (1), 74.

Humphris G., Kaney S., Broomfield D., Bayley T., Lilley J. (1994) *Stress in Junior Hospital Medical and Dental Staff.* Liverpool: University of Liverpool and Mersey Regional Health Authority.

Hyman R. (1988) Flexible specialisation: miracle or myth? In R. Hyman and W. Streeck (editors), *New Technology and Industrial Relations.* Oxford: Blackwell.

Ineson A. and Thom D. (1985) TNT Poisoning and the employment of women in the First World War. In P. Weindling (editor), *The Social History of Occupational Medicine*. London: Croom Helm.

Ingham G. (1967) Organisational size, orientations to work and industrial behaviour. *Sociology* 1, 239–258.

International Labour Office (1981) *The Effects of Technological and Structural Changes on the Employment and Working Conditions of Non–Manual Workers*. Geneva: ILO.

International Labour Office (1983) *New Technologies: The Impact On Employment and the Working Environment*. Geneva: ILO.

Israel B.A., Shurman J.J. and House J.J. (1989) Action research on occupational stress. *International Journal of Health Services* 19 (1), 135–155.

Jaffe E. (1986) Nationally speaking–the role of occupational therapy in disease prevention and health promotion. *American Journal of Occupational Therapy, Special Issue on Health Promotion* 40 (11), 749–752.

Jessop B. (1990) Regulation theories in retrospect. *Economy and Society* 19, 153–216.

Jessop B. (1991) The welfare state in the transition from fordism to post Fordism. In B. Jessop, H. Kastendiek, K. Neilsen and O.K. Pedersen (editors), *The Politics of Flexibility: Restructuring State and Industry in Britain, Germany and Scandinavia*. London: Edward Elgar.

Jette M. (1979) The standardised test of fitness in occupational health: a pilot project. *Canadian Journal of Public Health* 69, 431–438.

Johnson J. (1980) *Work Fragmentation, Human Degradation and Occupational Stress*. Mimeograph. Baltimore, MD: John Hopkins University.

Johnson J.V. (1991) Control, collectivity and the psychosocial work environment. In S. Sauter, J. Hurrell and C. Cooper (editors), *Job Control and Worker Health*. London: Wiley.

Johnson J.V. and Hall E.M. (1988) Job strain, work place social support and cardiovascular disease: a cross sectional study of a random sample of the swedish working population. *American Journal of Public Health* 78, 1336–1342.

Johnson J.V. and Johansson G. (1991) *Work Organisation, Occupational Health and Social Change*. New York: Baywood Publishing.

Kahn R. (1964) *Organisational Stress: Studies in Role Conflict and Ambiguity*. Chichester: Wiley.

Kahn R. and Weiss R. (1960) Definitions of work and occupation. *Social Problems* 8, 142–151.

Kahn R.L., Wolfe D.M., Quinn R.P., Snoek J.D. and Rosenthal R.A. (1964) *Organisational Stress*. New York: Wiley.

Kanter R.M. (1983) Managing transitions in organisational culture: the case of participative management at honeywell. In John R. Kimberely and Robert Quinn (editors), *New Futures: The Challenges of Managing Corporate Transitions*. Homewood, IL: Dow Jones-Irwin, pp. 195–217.

Karasek R. (1976) *The Impact of the Work Environment of Life Outside the Job*. Doctoral thesis, Massachusetts Institute of Technology.

Karasek R. (1979) Job demands, job decision latitude and mental strain: implications for job redesign. *Administrative Science Quarterly* 24, June, 285–308.

Karasek R. (1988) Job characteristics in relation to the prevalence of myocardial infarction in the US. HES and HANES. *American Journal of Public Health* 78, 910–918.

Karasek R. and Theorell T. (1990) *Healthy Work: Job Stress, Productivity and the Reconstruction of Working Life.* New York: Basic Books.

Karnell Corn J. (1992) *Response to Occupational Health Hazards: A Historical Perspective.* Van Nostrand Reinhold.

Kirwan M. and Armstrong D. (1995) Investigation of burn out in a sample of British general practitioners. *British Journal of General Practice* 45 (394), 259–260.

Kizer W. (1987) *The Healthy Workplace: A Blueprint for Corporate Action.* New York: Wiley.

Kleiner R.J. and Parker S. (1963) Goal striving, social status and mental disorder. *American Social Review* 28, 189–203.

Knights D. (1989) *Culture, Control and Competition.* Paper Presented at the PICT Workshop. University of Manchester Institute of Science and Technology, March 1989.

Knox S., Theorell T., Svensson J. and Waller D. (1985) The relation of social support and working environment to medical variables associated with elevated blood pressure in young males: a structural model. *Social Science and Medicine* 21, 525–531.

Kohn M. and Schooler C. (1983) *Work and Personality.* Norwood, NJ: Albex.

Kornhauser A. (1965) *Mental Health of the New Industrial Workers.* New York: Wiley.

Kritsikis S.P., Heinemann A.L. and Eitner S. (1968) The correlation of biological, psychological and sociological situations with agina pectoris. *Deutsch Gesundheit* 23, 1878–1885.

La Croix A.Z. and Haynes S.G. (1984) *Occupational Exposure to High Demand/Low Control Work and Coronary Heart Disease Incidence in the Framingham Cohort.* Paper presented at the Seventh Annual Meeting of the Society for Epidemiological Research, Houston. *American Journal of Epidemiology* 120, 341.

La Croix A.Z. and Haynes S.G. (1987) Gender differences in the health effects of workplace roles. In R. Barnett and G. Baruch (editors), *Gender and Stress.* New York: Macmillan, pp. 122–141.

La Rocco J.M., House J.S. and French J.R.P. (1980) Social support, occupational stress and health. *Journal of Health and Social Behaviour* 21, 202–218.

Lacey H.M. (1979) Perceived control and the methodological role of cognitive constructs. In Lawrence C. Perlmuter and R.A. Monty (editors), *Choice and Perceived Control.* Hillsdale, NJ: Lawrence Erlbaum Associates.

Lalonde M. (1974) *A New Perspective on the Health of Canadians.* Ottawa: Information Canada.

Lane C. (1989) *Management and Labour in Europe.* Aldershot, UK: Edward Elgar.

Lawrence P.R. and Lorsch J.W. (1967) *Organisational and Environment.* Cambridge, MA: Harvard University Press.

Lee R. and Lawrence P. (1985) *Organisational Behaviour: Politics at Work.* London: Hutchinson.

Lefcourt H.M. (1973) *Locus of Control–Current Trends in Theory and Research.* New York: Wiley.

Lennerlof L. (1989) Learning at work. In H. Kohnbluh and H. Leymann (editors), *Learning and Socialisation at the Workplace*. Stockholm: Prisma.

Levitan S.A. and Johnson C.M. (1982) *Second Thoughts on Work*. Kalamazoo: W.E. Upjohn Institute for Employment Research.

LFS (1996) *Labour Force Survey*. London: Stationery Office.

Lilijefors I. and Rahe R.H. (1970) An identical twin study of psychosocial factors in coronary heart disease in Sweden. *Psychosomatic Medicine* 32 (5), 525–543.

Lovering J. (1990) A perfunctory sort of post fordism: economic restructuring and labour market segmentation in Britain in the 1980s. *Work, Employment and Society* Special Issue May, 9–28.

Lysgaard S. (1960) *Workers Collectivity*. Oslo: University Forlaget.

Magnusson M. and Nilsson C. (1979) *To Work At Inconvenient Working Hours*. Stockholm: Prisma.

Makk L., Creech J., Whalen J. and Johnson M. (1974) Liver damage and angiosarcoma in vinyl chloride workers: a systematic detection program. *Journal of the American Medical Association* 230, 64–68.

Marcson S. (1970) *Automation, Alienation and Anomie*. New York: Harper and Row.

Marcuse H. (1972) *One Dimensional Man*. London: Abacus.

Margione T.H. (1973) The meaning of 'work': a matter of language. In R.P. Quinn and T.W. Margione (editors), *The 1969–1970 Survey of Working Conditions*, Chapter 7. Ann Arbor, MI: University of Michigan.

Margolis B.L., Kroes W.H. and Quinn R.P. (1974) Job stress: an unlisted occupational hazard. *Journal of Occupational Medicine* 16 (10), 654–661.

Marks R.U. (1967) Social stress and cardiovascular disease. *The Milbank Memorial Fund Quarterly* XLV (2), 51–107.

Marmot M. and Theorell T. (1988) Social class and cardiovascular disease: the contribution of work. *International Journal of Health Services* 18 (4), 659–673.

Martin R. and Fryer R.H. 91975) The deferential worker. In M. Bulmer (editor), *Working Class Images of Society*. London: Routledge and Kegan Paul.

Maslow A.H. (1943) A theory of human motivation. *Psychological Review* 50 (4), July, 370–396.

Mayo E. (1945) *The Social Problems of an Industrial Civilisation*. Cambridge, MA: Harvard University Press.

McDonaugh J.R., Hames C.G., Stulb S.C. and Garrison G.E. (1965) Coronary heart disease among negroes and whites in Evans County Georgia. *Journal of Chronic Disease* 18, 443–468.

McGregor D. (1987) *The Human Side of Enterprise*. London: Penguin.

McKevitt C., Morgan M, Simpson J. and Holland W.W. (1996) *Doctors' Health and Needs for Services*. London: Nuffield Provincial Hospitals Trust.

Meek J. (1993) An analysis of comprehensive health promotion programs' consistency with the systems model of health. *American Journal of Health Promotion* 17 (6), 336–342.

Meerbow L. and Page S. (1998) Getting the job done: emotion management and cardiopulmonary resuscitation in nursing. In G. Bendelow and S.J. Williams (editors), *Emotions in Social Life: Critical Themes and Contemparary Issues*. London: Routledge.

Meissner M. (1971) The long arm of the job. *Industrial Relations* 10: 238–260.

Menzies R., Tamblyn R., Farrant J.P., Hanley J. and Nunes F. (1993) The effect of varying levels of outdoor air supply on the symptoms of sick building syndrome. *New England Journal of Medicine* 328, 821–822; 877–878.

Merewether E.R.A. (1946) Industrial health. In *Annual Report of The Chief Inspector of Factories for the Year 1945*. London: HMSO, pp. 58–85.

Mettlin C. (1976) Occupational careers and the prevention of coronary prone behaviour. *Social Science and Medicine* 10, 367–372.

Meyer J.W. and Rowan B. (1977) Institutionalised organisations: formal structure as myth and ceremony. *American Journal of Sociology* 83, 340–361.

Miller J.G. (1960) Information input overload and psychopathy. *American Journal of Psychiatry* 8, 116.

Mills C.W. (1951) *White Collar: The American Middle Classes*. New York: OUP.

Mintzberg H. (1973) *The Nature of Managerial Work*. New York: Harper and Row.

Mintzberg H. (1975) The manager's job: folklore and fact. *Harvard Business Review* 53 (4), 49–61.

Mitchell D., Ledingham J. and Ashley-Miller M. (1996) *Taking Care of Doctors' Health*. London: Nuffield Provincial Hospitals Trust.

Morris J.N., Everitt M.G., Pollard R. and Chave S.P.W. (1980) Vigorous exercise in leisure time, protection against coronary heart disease. *Lancet* (ii) 1207–1210.

Mullins L.J. (1994) *Management and Organisational Behaviour*, third edition. London: Pitman Publishing.

National Heart, Lung and Blood Institute (1980) National High Blood Pressure Education Program At Mass Mutual: *Offsite Care and Good Monitoring Reduce Medical Costs, Re: High Blood Pressure Control in the Work Setting*. Bethsheda, MD: National Heart, Lung and Blood Institute.

Navarro V. (1976) The underdevelopment of health of working america, causes, consequences and possible solutions. In *Medicine Under Capitalism*. New York: Prodist, pp. 82–99.

Navarro V. (1980) Work ideology and science: the case of medicine. *International Journal of Health Services* 10 (4), 523–550.

Navarro V. (1982) The labour process and health: a historical materialist interpretation. *International Journal of Health Services* 12 (1), 5–29.

Navarro V. (1985) US Marxist scholarship in the analysis of health and medicine. *International Journal of Health Services* 15 (4), 525–545.

Navarro V. and Berman D. (1983) *Health and Work Under Capitalism*. Farmingdale, NY: Baywood Press.

Neff W.S. (1968) *Work and Human Behaviour*. New York: Wiley.

Nelson D., Sennett L., Lefebvre R., Loiselle L., McClements L. and Carleton R. (1987) A campaign strategy for weight loss at worksites. *Health Education Research, Special Issue: Health Promotion in Work Settings* 2 (1), 27–32.

Nichols T. (1990) Industrial safety in Britain and the 1974 Health and Safety At Work Act: the case of manufacturing. *International Journal of Sociology and Law* 18, 317–342.

O'Donnell M.P. and Ainsworth T. (1984) *Health Promotion in the Workplace*. New York: Wiley.

O'Donnell M.P. and Harris J. (1994) *Health Promotion in the Workplace*. New York: Wiley.

Ollman B. (1971) *Alienation: Marx's Concept of Man in Capitalist Society.* Cambridge, MA: Cambridge University Press.

Opel G.L. and Clark M.W. (1988) Sport, fitness and recreation in the Japanese workplace. In E.F. Bloom, R.A. Clumper, B.B. Pendleton and C.A. Pooley (editors), *Comparative Physical Education and Sport,* Vol. 5. New York and London: Human Kinetic Books, pp. 285–292.

OSHA (1974) *New Standard for Vinyl Chloride. Job Safety and Health.* US Department of Labour.

Ouchi W.G. (1981) *Theory Z: How American Business Can Meet the Japanese Challenge.* Reading, MA: Addison Wesley.

Ouchi W.G. (1983) Organisational culture. *Annual Review of Sociology* 11, 457–483.

Paffenbarger R.S. and Hale W.E. (1975) Work activity and coronary heart mortality. *The New England Journal of Medicine* 292 (11), 545–550.

Palloix C. (1980) *Process Production and Crises Under Capitalism.* New York: Blume Ediciones.

Palmore E. (1969) Predicting longevity: a follow–up controlling for age. *Gerontologist* 9 (4), 247–250.

Pantry S. (1995) *Occupational Health.* London: Chapman and Hall.

Parker S. and Kleiner R.J. (1966) *Mental Illness in the Urban Negro Community.* New York: The Free Press.

Parkinson R. (1982) *Managing Health Promotion in the Workplace.* Palo Alto, CA: Mayfield.

Parsons T. (1955) *Family, Socialisation and Interaction Process.* New York: The Free Press.

Patty F.A. (1962) *Industrial Hygiene and Toxicology,* second edition, Vol. 2. New York: Wiley, pp. 1303–1304.

Paul O. (1963) A longitudinal study of coronary heart disease. *Circulation* 28, 20–31.

Pearlin L. (1981) The stress process. *Journal of Health and Social Behaviour* 22, 337–356.

Pell S. and D'Alonzo C.A. (1958) Myocardial infarction in a one year study. *Journal of American Medical Association* 166, 332–337.

Pencak M. (1991) Workplace health promotion programmes. An overview. *Nursing Clinics of North America* 26 (1), 23–240.

Peters T.J. and Waterman R.H. (1982) In *Search of Excellence: Lessons from America's Best Run Companies.* New York: Harper and Row.

Pettigrew A.W. (1973) *The Politics of Organisational Decision Making.* London: Tavistock Publication.

Pheasant S. (1991) *Ergonomics, Work and Health.* London: MacMillan Press.

Poire M. and Sabel C. (1984) *The Second Industrial Divide.* New York: Basic Books.

Porter A.M.D., Howie J.G.R. and Levinson A. (1985) Measurement of stress as it effects the work of the general practitioner. *Family Practice* 2 (3), 136–146.

Porter L.W. and Lawler E.E. (1965) Properties of organisation structure in relation to job attitudes and job behaviour. *Psychology Bulletin* 64, 23–51.

Prange G.W. (1981) *At Dawn We Slept: The Untold Story of Pearl Harbour.* New York: McGraw–Hill.

Pringle R. (1988) *Secretaries Talk.* London: Verso.

Pugh D.S. and Hickson D.J. (1976) *Organisational Structure in its Context*. Farnborough: Saxon House.

Quine L. (1999) Workplace bullying in NHS community trust: staff questionnaire survey. *British Medical Journal* 318, 23rd January, 228–232.

Quinn R.P., Seashore S. and Mangione I. (1971) *Survey of Working Conditions*. Washington, DC: US Government Printing Office.

Ramazzini B. (1964) *De Morbis Artificum Diatriba /Diseases of Workers*. New York Academy of Medicine: Hafner Publishing Company.

Ratanen J. (1991) *Occupational Health Services in Europe*. Copenhagen: WHO.

Report of A Committe of Enquiry on Industrial Health Services ('*The Dale Committee*'). London: HMSO, 1951.

Rider B. and White V. (1986) Occupational therapy education in health promotion and disease prevention. *American Journal of Occupational Therapy Special Issue on Health Promotion* 40 (11), 781–783.

Robens Committee (1972) *Safety and Health at Work*. Cmnd., 5034. London: HMSO.

Roberts M.F., Wenger C.B., Stolwijk J.A.J. and Nadel E.R. (1977) Skin, blood flow and sweating changes following exercise training and heat acclimation. *Journal of Applied Physiology: Respiratory Environmental Exercise Physiology* 43, 133–137.

Roesthlisberger F.J. and Dickson W.J. (1939) *Management and The Worker*. Cambridge, MA: Harvard University Press.

Roethlisberger F.J. and Dickson W.J. (1950) *Management and the Worker*. Cambridge, MA: Harvard University Press.

Rose M. (1978) *Industrial Behaviour*. London: Penguin.

Rosen G. (1937) On the historical investigation of occupational diseases: an apercu. *Bulletin of the History of Medicine* 5, 941–946.

Rosen G. (1943) *History of Miners Diseases: A Medical and Social Interpretation*. New York: Science History.

Rosen R.H. (1984) Worksite health promotion: fact or fantasy? *Corporate Comment* 1, 1–8.

Rotter J.B. (1966) Generalized expectancies for internal versus external control for reinforcement. *Physiological Monograph of General Applied Studies*, No. 80, p. 609.

Rowntree & Co., Ltd. (1916) *Industrial Betterment at the Cocoa Works, York*.

Roy D. (1952) Quota restriction and gold bricking in a machine shop. *American Journal of Sociology* 57, 427–442.

Roy D. (1953) Work satisfaction and social reward in quota achievement. *American Sociological Review* 18, 507–514.

Roy D. (1954) Efficiency and the fix: informal intergroup relations in a piecework machine shop. *American Journal of Sociology* 60, 255–266.

Roy D. (1960) Banana time: job satisfaction and informal interaction. *Human Organisation* 18, 158–161.

Roy D. (1973) Banana time. In G. Salaman and K. Thompson (editors), *People and Organisations*. London: Longman.

Russek H.I. and Zohman B.L. (1958) Relative significance of heredity, diet and occupational stress in coronary heart disease in young adults. *American Journal of the Sciences* 235, 266–275.

Ryan G.A. and Brampton M. (1988) Comparison of data process operators with and without symptoms. *Community Health Studies* 12, 63–68.

Ryle J.A. and Russell W.T. (1949) The natural history of coronary disease: a clinical and epidemiological study. *British Heart Journal* 11, 370–389.

Salaman G. (1986) *Working*. London: Tavistock Publications.

Sales S. (1969) Organisation role as a risk factor in coronary disease. *Administrative Science Quarterly* 14, 325–336.

Sales S.M. and House J. (1971) Job dissatisfaction as a possible risk factor in coronary heart disease. *Journal of Chronic Disease* 23, 861–873.

Sathe V. (1985) *Culture and Related Corporate Realities*. Homewood, IL: Richard D. Irwin.

Sayer A. (1989) Post Fordism in question. *International Journal of Urban and Regional Research* 13, 666–695.

Sayles L.R. (1958) *Behaviour of Industrial Work Groups*. London: Wiley.

Schatzkin A. (1978) Health and labour power: a theoretical investigation. *International Journal of Health Services* 8, 213–233.

Schein E. (1981) Does Japanese management style have a message for American managers? *Sloan Management Review* 23, 55–68.

Schein E. (1983) The role of the founder in creating organisational culture. *Organisational Dynamics* Summer, 13–28.

Schein E. (1985) *Organisational Culture and Leadership*. San Francisco, CA: Jossey–Bass.

Schilling R. (1991) Occupational medicine for one and all. *British Journal of Industrial Medicine* 48, 445–450.

Schonberger R. (1982) Production workers bear major quality responsibility in Japanese industry. *Industrial Engineering* 14 (12), 34–40.

Schultz A.J., Israel B.A., Zimmerman M.A. and Checkonay B.N. (1995) *Empowerment as a Multi-level Construct: Perceived Control of the Individual, Organisational and Community Levels*. New York: Delmar.

Schwalbe M.L. and Staples C.L. (1986) Class position, work experience and health. *International Journal of Health Services* 16 (4), 583–602.

Seccombe I. and Ball J. (1992) *Back Injured Nurses: A Profile*. RCN Discussion Papers.

Seccombe I. and Buchan J. (1993) Absent nurses: the costs and consequences. *IMS (RCN) Report*, No. 250. Institute of Manpower Services.

Seedhouse D. (1991) *Health, the Foundations of Achievement*. Chichester: Wiley.

Selikoff I. and Culyer H.E. (1975) Toxicity of vinyl chloride and polyvinyl chloride. *Annals of the New York Academy of Sciences* 246.

Selznick P. (1949) *TVA and the Grass Roots*. Berkley, CA: University of California Press.

Shephard J.M. (1971) *Automation and Alienation*. Cambridge, MA: MIT Press.

Shirom A., Eden D., Silberwasser S. and Kellerman J.J. (1973) Job stresses and risk factors in coronary heart disease among occupational categories in kibbutzim. *Social Science and Medicine* 7, 875–892.

Shutzker P. (1985) Ergonomics in microelectronic office technology. *Occupational Health Nursing* 33 (12), 610–614.

Sievers B. (1984) Motivation as a surrogate for meaning. In M. Alvesson (editor), *Organisation Theory and Technocratic Consciousness*. Berlin: De Grutyer.

Silverman D. (1970) *Theory of Organisations*. London: Heinemann.

Simpson B. (1990) Environmental support for professional nursing practice. *Nurse to Nurse* 1 (5), October, 19–20.

Skrzycki C. (1988) *'Mommy Tack' Author Answers Her Many Critics*. Washington Post, March 19, Section C, p. 1.

Sorensen G., Stoddard A., Ockene J.K., Hunt M.K. and Youngstrom R. (1996) Worker participation in an integrated health promotion/health protection program: results from the Well Works Projects. *Health Education Quarterly* 23 (2), May, 191–203.

Springett J. and Dugdill L. (1995) Workplace health promotion programmes: towards a framework for education. *Health Education Quarterly* 54, 88–98.

Stalmer J., Kjelsberg M. and Hall Y. (1960) Epidemiologic studies of cardiovascular renal diseases: i. Analysis of mortality by age–race–sex–occupation. *Journal of Chronic Disease* 12, 440–455.

Sterner J. (1943) Determining margin of safety–criteria for defining a 'harmful' substance. *Journal of Industrial Medicine* 12, 514–518.

Stogdill R.M. and Coons A.E. (1957) *Leader Behaviour: Its Description and Measurement*. Research Monograph No. 88, Bureau of Business Research. Ohio, OH: The Ohio State University.

Sui G.H. (1971) Work and serenity. *Occupational and Mental Health* 1 (1), 10–16.

Sutherland I. (1987) *Health Education – Half A Policy: The Rise and Fall of Health Education Council*. London: NEC Publications.

Sutherland V.J. and Cooper C.L. (1992) Job stress, satisfaction and mental health among general practitioners before and after the introduction of the new contract. *British Medical Journal* 304, 1545–1548.

Svensson L. (1989) A democratic strategy for organisational change. *International Journal of Health Services* 19 (2), 319–334.

Syme S.L., Hyman M.M. and Enterline P.E. (1964) Some social and cultural factors associated with the occurrence of coronary heart disease. *Journal of Chronic Disease* 17, 277–289.

Tabor M. (1983) Worker health in the automated office. *Occupational Health and Safety* 52 (4), 22–26.

Taplin I.M. (1989) Segmentation and the organisation of work in the italian apparel industry. *Social Science Quarterly* 70, 408–424.

Taplin I.M. (1995) Flexible production, rigid jobs: lessons from the clothing industry. *Work and Occupations* 22 (4), November, 412–438.

Taskforce (1993) *The Health of the Nation*. Workplace Taskforce Report, September 1993.

Taylor F.W. (1947) *The Principles of Scientific Management* (originally published in 1911). London: Harper and Row.

Teleky L. (1948) *History of Factory and Mine Hygiene*. New York: Science History.

Tennan H., Gillen R. and Drum P.E. (1982) The debilitating effect of exposure to non contingent escape: a test of the learned helplessness model. *Journal of Personality* 50, 387–408.

Terryberry S. (1968) *The Organisation of Environments*. Phd Thesis, University Microfilms. Ann Arbor, MI: University of Michigan.

Theorell T. (1987) Psychosocial work conditions before myocardial infarction in young men. *International Journal of Cardiology* 15, 33–46.

Theorell R. and Rahe R.H. (1972) Behaviour and life satisfaction characteristics of swedish subjects with myocardial infarction. *Journal of Chronic Disorders* 25, 139.

Thompson P. and McHugh D. (1990) *Work Organisations*. London: MacMillan.

Thompson P. and Warhurst C. (1998) *Workplaces of the Future*. Basingstoke: MacMillan.

Trahair R.C.S. (1984) *The Humanist Temper: The Life and Work of Elton Mayo*. New Brunswick, NJ: Transaction Books.

Trice H.M. and Belasco J. and Alutto J.A. (1969) The role of ceremonials in organisational behaviour. *Industrial and Labour Relations Review* 23rd October, 40–51.

Trice H.M. and Beyer J.M. (1984) Studying organisational cultures through rites and ceremonial. *Academy of Management Review* 9 (4), 653–659.

Trice H.M. and Beyer J.M. (1991) Cultural leadership in organisations. *Organisation Science* 2 (2), 149–169.

Trice H.M. and Roman P.M. (1971) Occupational risk factors in mental health and the impact of role change experiences. In J. Leedy (editor), *Compensation in Psychiatric Disability and Rehabilitation*. Springfield, IL: Chas C. Thomas, pp. 145–204.

Triolo P. (1989) Occupational health hazards of hospital staff nurses. Part 1: Overview and psychosocial stressors. *Journal of the American Academy of Occupational Health Nursing* 37 (6), June, 232–237.

Trist E. and Banfort K.W. (1951) Some social and psychological consequences of the long wall method of coal cutting. *Human Relations* February, 3–38.

TUC (1924) The waste of capitalism. In Milne Bailey (editor), *Trade Union Documents*. 1929, pp. 67–70.

Turner B.A. (1971) *Exploring The Industrial Subculture*. London: MacMillan Press.

Tyrer F.H. and Lee K. (1982) *Occupational Health*. London: Wright.

Tyrer F.H. and Lee K. (1984) *A Synopsis of Occupational Medicine*, first edition. London: Wright.

US Department of Health and Human Services (1993) 1992 National survey of worksite health promotion activities: summary. *American Journal of Health Promotion* 7, 452–464.

Veterans (1970) Results in patients with diastolic blood pressures averaging 90 through 114 mmHg. *Journal of the American Medical Association* 213, 1143–1152.

Veterans (1972) Effects in the treatment on morbidity in hyperstension IV. Influence of age, diastolic pressure and poor cardiovascular disease: further analysis of side effects. *Circulation* 45, 991–1004.

Veterans Co-operative Administration (1967) Effects on morbidity in hypertension, results in patients with diastolic blood pressures averaging 15 through 129 mmHg. *Journal of the American Medical Association* 202, 1028–1034.

Viola P.L., Bigotti A. and Caputo A. (1971) Oncogenic response of rat skin lungs and bones to vinyl chloride. *Cancer Research* 31, 516–519.

Virchow R. (1879) *Gesammelte Abhandhugen as den Gebret der oeffentlichen Medizin und der Seuchenlehre*, Vol. 1. Berlin: Hirschwald, pp. 305, 321–334.

Volpert W. (1986) Mental regulation of work behaviour. In J. Rutenfranz and U. Kleinbeck (editors), *Encyclopaedia of Psychology*. Gottingen: Hogrefe.

von Bertalanffy L. (1951) Problems of general systems theory: a new approach to the unity of science. *Human Biology* 23, 302–312.

Waitzkin H. (1981) The social origins of illness: a neglected history. *International Journal of Health Services* 11 (1), 77–103.

Waldron H.A. (1996) Occupational health during the Second World War: hope deferred or hope abandoned? *Medical History* 41, 197–212.

Walker C.R. (1952) *The Man on the Assembly Line*. Cambridge, MA: Harvard University Press.

Walsh D.C., Jennings S., Margione T. and Merrigan D. (1991) Health promotion versus health protection? Employee perceptions and concerns. *Journal of Public Health Policy* 12, 148–164.

Walters D.R. (1990) *Worker Participation in Health and Safety: A European Comparison*. London: Institute of Employment Rights.

Walters D.R. and Gourlay S. (1990) *Statutory Employee Involvement in Health and Safety at the Workplace: A Report of the Implementation and Effectiveness of the Safety Representatives and Safety Committees Regulation 1977*. Contract Research Report No. 20/1990. London: HMSO.

Walton R. (1985) The management of interdepartmental conflict: a model and review. *Administrative Science Quarterly* 14, 73–84.

Wardell W.I., Hyman M.M. and Bahnson C.B. (1964) Stress and coronary disease in three field studies. *Journal of Chronic Disease* 17, 73–84.

Wedderburn D. and Crompton R. (1972) *Workers Attitudes and Technology*. Cambridge, MA: Cambridge University Press.

Weindling P. (1985) *Social History of Occupational Health*. London: CroomHelm.

Weinstein M. (1986) Lifestyle, stress and work: strategies for health promotion. *Health Promotion* 1 (3), 363–371.

Westgaard R.H. and Aaras A. (1984) Postural muscle strain as a causal factor in the development of musculoskeletal illness. *Applied Ergonomics* 15, 162–174.

Westgaard R.H. and Aaras A. (1985) The effect of improved workplace design on the environment of work related musculoskeletal illness. *Applied Ergonomics* 16, 91–97.

Westlander G. (1976) *Working Conditions and the Content of Leisure*. Stockholm: Swedish Council for Personal Administration.

Wheen F. (1998) G2. *The Guardian*, p. 5.

WHO (1946) *Constitution*. Geneva: WHO.

WHO (1981) Development indicators for monitoring progress towards health for all by the year 2000. In *Health for All Series*, No. 4. Geneva: WHO.

WHO (1984) *Health Promotion: A Discussion Document on the Concepts and Principles*. Copenhagen: WHO.

WHO (1988a) *Health Promotion for Working Populations*. Technical Report Services 765. Geneva: WHO.

WHO (1988b) *Health Systems Research in Action: Case Studies, Programme on Health Systems Research and Development*. Division of Strengthening of Health Services. Geneva: WHO.

Whyte W.F. (1948) *Human Relations in the Restaurant Industry*. New York. McGraw–Hill.

Wilkins A.L. and Ouchi W.G. (1983) Efficient cultures: exploring the relationship between culture and organisational performance. *Administrative Science Quarterly* 28, 468–481.

Wilkinson C. (1997) *Managing Health at Work: a Guide for Managers and Workplace Health Specialists*. London: Chapman and Hall.

Wilkinson C. (1999) Management, the workplace and health promotion: fantasy or reality? *Health Education Journal* 58, March, 56–65.

Williams J.L. (1961) *Accidents and Illness at Work*. London: Staples.

Willis E. (1986) RSI as a social process. *Community Health Studies* 10, 210–219.

Winefield H.R. and Anstey T.J. (1991) Job stress in general practice: practitioner age, sex and attitudes as predictors. *Family Practice* 8, 140–144.

Wolf S. (1969) Psychosocial forces in myocardial infarction and sudden death. *Circulation* 40 (Supplement 4), 74–83.

Wolinsky F.D. (1988) *The Sociology of Health: Principles, Practitioners and Issues*, second edition. Belmont, CA: Wadsworth.

Womack J.P., Jones D.T., Roos D. (1990) *The Machine that Changed the World*. New York: Harper.

Wood S. (1993) The Japanization of Fordism. *Economic and Industrial Democracy* 14, 535–555.

Woodward J. (1958) *Management and Technology*. London: HMSO.

Woodward J. (1980) *Industrial Organisation: Theory and Practice*. London: Oxford University Press.

Wynne R. (1994) *Workplace Health Promotion – A Specification for Training*. European Foundation for the Improvement of Living and Working Conditions. WP/94/22/EN.

Wynne R. and Clarkin N. (1992) *Under Construction, Building for Health in the EC Workplace*. Dublin: European Foundation for the Improvement of Living and Working Conditions.

Zadjow G. (1995) Caring and nurturing in the lives of women married to alcoholics. *Women's Studies International Forum* 18, 535–546.

Zaleznik A., Ondrack J. and Silver A. (1970) Social class, occupation and mental illness. In A. McLean (editor), *Mental Health and Work Organizastions*. Chicago, IL: Rand McNally.

Zucker L.G. (1977) The role of institutionalisation in cultural persistence. *American Sociological Review* 42, 726–743.

Index

Aaras, A. 11
ability to unwind 9
absence 2, 5, 62
accidents 1, 40; prevention 44
action 81
Adams, A. 92
Adams, J.S. 5
Aglietta, M. 103
Agricola 25
Akerstedt, T., 20
alcohol 35
Aldridge, J.T. 29
alienation 12, 113
Alienation and Mental Health 117
Allsop 78
angina pectoris 22
anomie 79; anomie human relations
    theory 79
Anstey, T.J. 21
anxiety 6
Arendt, H. 7, 75, 80
Argyris, C. 22, 92, 125
Argyropoulos-Grisanos 78
Armstrong, D. 21
Aronowitz, S. 15
Arthur, R.J. 18
Asbestosis 59
asthma 59
Atkinson, J. 102
authoritarian leadership 109, 118
autonomous groups 158
Averill, J.R. 16

Bainton, C.R. 22
Baker, F. 144 166
Ball, J. 21
Bampton, M. 12

Battiscombe, G. 28
Beaumont 78
Beckhard, R. 99
behaviour 3
Belcher, J. 21
Berkson, D. 22
Berman, D. 12
Betera, R.I. 149, 151, 164
Beyer, J.M. 95, 100
Beynon, H. 79
Black, D. 69
Blanchard, K. 2
Blauner, R. 7, 93, 118
BMA 51
boredom 117
Bosch, G. 104
Boumans, N.P.G. 2
Bowey, A. 94
Bowles, S. 78
Bradley, G. 23
Braverman, H. 78, 161
Breslow, L. 20, 22, 146
Breuker, 162
Britain 26, 55; infrastructure 149;
    position in workplace health
    promotion 148
Brown, I. 23
Buchan, J. 21
Buck, V. 23
Buell, P. 20, 22
bullying 6
Bulmer, M. 79
Bunt, 163
Burawoy, M. 79
Burns, T. 93
Burrell, G. 100 101
business planning 144

cancer 43, 59
capitalism 35, 102
Caplan, R. 14, 21, 22
care 152
Cassell, J. 16
Caudhill, W. 96
Chadwick, 29, 32
Chadwickian tradition 32
Chambers, R. 21
changing nature of work 102
characteristics of industrial society 76
CHD 14
chemicals 59
Child, J. 94
children 29; child like behaviour 125
civil servants 16
Clarkin, N. 164
class 8; position 15
Cleland, L.G. 11
Clutterbuck, R.C. 43, 102
Coburn, D. 12, 77
codetermination 158
Cohen, B.H. 77
Cohen, D. 150
COMA 79
Committee Enquiry 51
compartmentalisation 109
components of the workplace 2
concepts of health 7
conflict 108
Conrad, P. 144, 158
Conrad, R. 12, 19
contemporary theories 94
contribution of the trades unions 43
control 9, 16; destiny 16
Coons, A.E. 2
Cooper, C.L. 10, 21, 22, 144
Cooper, R. 100
Coren, A. 12
coronary heart disease 9
Cotgrove, S. 78
Cousens 58
criticisms 79
Crompton, R. 78
CSO 1995 163
Culyer, H.E. 77
Cunningham 58

D'Alonzo, C.A. 22
Dalton, M. 96
dangerous conditions of work 147;
    death 25, 79

Davidson, R. 2
Dawson, S. 2
De Man, H. 7 87
Deal, T.E. 97, 99
decision latitude 10
defining work 75
degradation 118
democratic working 135, 138, 142;
    democratico-participatory approach
    144, 158
Denison, D.R. 99
Department of Employment 1993 163
Department of Health 1998 70
depression 6
Derrida, J. 100
deskilling 9, 111
determinants of workplace health 9
Dickens 138, 139
Dickson, W.J. 86, 123
disability 12
discrimination 159
disease 40, 59; prevention 160
dissatisfaction 123
division of labour 80, 82
Drucker, P.F. 84
Dubin, R. 78
Dugdill, L. 149, 164
Durkheim, E. 75, 79
Dwr Cymru, HPW 160
dysfunctional organisation 3

Eddy, J.M. 164
Edwards 161
effect of capitalism 108
elements of organisational culture 99
Ellenborg 26
emerging perspectives on workplace
    health promotion 145
Emerson, R.M. 85
emotion work 9
employee 70
employers 70
Engellian society 36
Engels, F. 2, 35
Engelstad 134
environment 4
equality 121
European Commission 104, 166
European Framework Directive 56
European links 56
European Network for Workplace
    Health Promotion 167

European Union 68
evaluation 164
expropriation 109
Eyer, J. 77, 78

factory 27; Acts 29; doctors 30;
    inspectors 30
Fairburn, J. 153
fairness 121
family 40; work demands 167
Fayol, H. 85
fear 129
Feilding, J., 144, 145, 146, 148
Feildstein, A. 153
Feinleib, M. 127
feminist perspective 38
Ferguson, D.A. 11
Fineman, 10
Firth-Cozens, J. 21
Fischer, S. 16
flexibility 139; flexible labour market
    102
Forslin 119
Fortes, M. 3, 100
Foucault, M. 7, 101
fragmentation 110; fragmented and
    constrained work 118
Frankenhauser, M. 9, 16, 117
Freidmann, F.A. 75, 78
French, J.R.P. 14, 22, 119
Freund, 1998 9
Friedlander 1967 78, 1966 119
Friend, B. 154
Frith, H. 9
frustration 5, 13; powerlessness 17
Fry, 1988 11
Fryer, R.H. 79

Gallie, D. 78
Gardell, B. 9, 10, 12, 16, 78, 114 134
Gardener, B.B. 96
Garfield, J. 12, 13, 77
Garfinkel, H. 3, 100
gender 8, 103
general practitioner 56
Gephart, R.J. 3
Gerhardt, U. 8
Germany 59
Giddens, A. 77
Gillespie, R. 86
Ginsburg, N. 56
Gintis, H. 78

Glasgow, R.E. 148, 153
Goldenhar, L.M. 152
Goldstein, K. 90
Goldthorpe, J.H. 79
Gorz, A. 77
Gottleib, N. 144
Gourlay, S. 44
government 55, 69
Green, G.M. 144, 166
Greenhow, E.H. 28
Lord Gregson 55
Grieco, A. 11
Grint, K. 120
Grossman, R. 144
group pressures 2
guardian, 64
Guest 93
Gunderson, E.K. 18
Gustavsen, B. 18, 19, 78, 114

Hagberg, M. 19
Hall, E. 9, 12, 14, 127
Handy, C. 97
Hansaari Model 153–154
harassment 6
Harris, J. 152
Harrison, R. 97
Havighurst, R.J. 75
Hawkin 78
Hawthorne Effect 86
Haycox, A. 150
Haynes, S. 127
hazards at work 54, 63
HEA 1997 156
health 1, 8; education 143; health and
    safety 44; Health and Safety at Work
    Act 1974 47; Health and Safety
    Executive 68; Health of the Nation
    Taskforce 53; improvement 24, 50,
    68, 115; link between health
    promotion and occupational health
    in Britain 151; problems 63;
    promotion 25, 138, 141, 163;
    propaganda 34; protection 144; risk
    56; schemes 43; surveillance 57
health–illness dichotomy 4
heart disease. 14
Henry, J. 96
Hersey, P. 2
Hertzberg, F. 78, 92
hierarchy 15; class and control 15;
    hierarchical division 23, 109; needs 5

Hikson, D.J. 93
Hirst, P. 102
historical context 25
Hochschild, A.R. 10
Hofstede, G. 98
Hoggett, P. 102
HoN Taskforce 156
House, J. 19
HPW 144
HSE 24, 67, 153, 163
Hugentobler, M.K. 164
human needs 74; humanism of labour 82
Humphris, G. 21
Hyman, R. 103

illness 1, 56
ILO 23
impact on worker health 113
individual lifestyle and behavioural
    change 145
industry 38; accidents 36; conflict 80;
    health 41; production 121; revolution
    26
inequalities 5, 9, 36; in health 69
influences of work on states of mind 88
Ingham, G. 78
injury 10
instinct 88
insurance 42
isolation 120
Israel, B.A. 164
issues: accountability 62; limitations 157

Jaffe, E. 144
Jessop, B. 102, 104
job dissatisfaction 14, 18; satisfaction 6,
    124
Johansson, G. 114 158
Johnson, J.V. 9, 10, 12, 114, 117, 158
Joy in Work 87

Kahn, R. 21, 23, 75
Kannel, W. 127
Karasek, J. 78
Karasek, R. 9, 10, 16
Karlsson, 1985 161
Karnell Corn, J. 148
Kennedy, A.A. 97, 99
Kirwan, M. 21
Kitzinger, C. 9
Kizer, W. 144
Kleiner, R.J. 18

Knights, D. 100
knowledge 169
Knox, S. 23
Kohn, M. 19
Kompier 165
Kornhauser, A. 11, 119
Kritskis, S.P. 11

La Croix, A.Z. 127
La Rocco, J.M. 12
labour 75; labour process 112; labouring
    80
Labour government 68
lace making 37
Lacey, H.M. 16
lack of autonomy 19
Lalonde, M. 141
Landeweerd, J.A. 2
Lane, C. 102
Larwence, P.R. 93
Lawler, E.E. 1965 14
Lawrence, P. 94
lead poisoning 38
leadership 99
Lee, K. 47
Lee, R. 94
Lefcourt, H.M. 16
legislation 1, 44
leisure 77
Lennerlof, L. 125
Levi 165
LFS 105
lifestyle 152; risk factor 159
Lilijefors, I. 19
Lockwood, D. 79
Look After Your Heart (LAYH) 148
Look After Yourself (LAY) 148
Lorsch, J.W. 93
loss of freedom 117
Lovering, J. 103
Luxembourg declaration 141
Lysgaard, S. 123

machine-pacing 10
Magnusson, M. 20
Makk, L. et al 77
managers 3
Marcson, 1970 11
Marcuse, H. 77
Margione, T.H. 75
Margolis, B.L. 14
Marks, R.U. 22

Marmot, M. 10, 17
Martin, R. 79
Marxian 2
Marxist 12
Maslow, A.H. 5
Mayo 86, 96
McDonough, J.R. 22
McGettigan, J. 153
McGregor, D. 91
McKevitt, C. 21
McLeroy, K.R. 144
Meager, N. 102
meaningful work 118, 119
means of labour 112
medical model of health 1
medical profession 8
Meek, J. 153
Meerbow, L. 9
Meissner, M. 18
mental health 11
Menzies, R. 1993 153
Merewether, E.R.A. 51
Mettlin, C. 15
Miller, J.G. 15
Mills, C.W. 78
Mintzberg, H. 96
missed opportunities 51
Mitchell, D. 13
Morals of Apprentices Act 1802 27
motivation 5
MRC 51
Mullins, L.J. 21
multilevel approach to health
    improvement 144, 157
multiple sites 67
musculo-skeletal disorders 19, 23
myocardial infarction 22

National Heart, Lung and Blood
    Institute 147
nature of work 74, 87
Navarro, V. 4, 12, 77
negroes 22
Nelson, D. 1987 144
neo-human relations school 90
NHS 21, 54
Nichols, T. 44
Nilsson, C. 20
normality 101
Nursing 57

occupation 76

occupational health 25; conditions 12;
    development 45; nurses 57; services
    46
occupational hygienist 59
occupational medicine 42
occupational physicians 57
occupational safety and health
    legislation 29
O'Donnell, M.P. 152
Office of National Statistics 163
Oldenburg, 1995 148
Ollman, B. 77
organisation of production. 79
organisational approach 144, 157;
    behaviour 3; culture 22, 95;
    ideologies 97
OSH 153
OSHA 77
Ottawa Charter 140
Ouchi, W.G. 99
Our Healthier Nation 69
Owen, R. 27

Page, S. 9
Palloix, C. 78
Palmore, E. 18
Pantry, S. 144
Paracelsus, 25
Parker, S. 18
Parkinson, R. 144
Parsons, T. 8
participation 9
passivity 117
Patty, F.A. 77
Pearlin, L. 77
Peel, 29
Pell, S. 22
Pencak, M. 144
perception of health promotion in
    Britain 151
performance 2
personal say, personal control 119
Peters, T.J. 98
Peterson, D.R. 22
Pettigrew, A.W. 96
Pheasant, S. 2
physical and mental demands 19
planning 169
Poire, M. 102
policies 7
political organisation 94
political reform 128

politics 4, 76
polyvinyl chloride 43
poor work conditions 9, 27
Poor Law Commission 32
Porter, A.M.D. 21
Porter, L.W. 14
post-Fordism 102
Post-modernist paradigms 100
pottery industry 38
poverty 8, 36
power 15
powerlessness 13, 118
Prange, G.W. 3
prevention 56, 152
Pringle, R. 64
private and public domain 127
production 102
proletarianisation 110
psychological distress 12; issues 135;
    violence 65
public health 32, 41
Pugh, D.S. 93
punishments 8

quality of working life 9
quantitative and qualitative overload 14
Quine, L. 6, 13
Quinn, R.P. 14
Qvale 134

race 8, 103
Rahe, R.H. 19
Ramazzini, B. 2, 26
Ratanen, J. 153
recent regulatory developments 63
reformers 27
regulation of factories 30
rehabilitation 57
repetitive strain injuries 11
Rider, B. 144
rights and ceremonials 3
rights of degradation 3
risk 60; assessment 63
Robens Committee 52
Lord Robens 47
Roberts, M.F. 77
Roethlisberger, F.J. 86, 123
role: overload 13; underload 13;
    relationships 21
Roman, P.M. 3, 100
Rose, M. 84
Rosen, G. 41

Rotter, J.B. 77
Rowntree, 33
Roy, D. 94, 96
RSI 12
Russek, H.I. 13
Russell, W.T. 22
Ryan, G.A. 12
Ryle, J.A. 22

Sabel, C. 102
safety 42
Sales, S.M. 14
Sales, S.M. 19
SANE approach 161
Sathe, V. 97
satisfaction 74
Sayer, A. 103
Sayles, L.R. 93
Scala, K. 144
Scandinavia 59
Scandinavian school of workplace
    health 19
Schatzkin, A. 12
Schein, E. 22, 98
Schilling, R. 144
Schooler, C. 19
Schulte, P.A. 152
Schwalbe M.L. 12
Seccombe, I. 21
Seedhouse, D. 8
self esteem 114
Selikoff, I. 77
Selznick, P. 96
Lord Shaftesbury 28
Shephard, J.M. 11
shift work 10
Shirom, A. 22
Shultz, A.J. 144
sick organisation 2, 5
sickness 2, 4, 24
Sievers, B. 86
Sigerist, H. 41
Silverman, D. 94, 98
Sind 134
sisyphus complex, 17
skill 9; discretion 120
Skrzycki, C. 127
Slutzker 24
social causes of ill health 71
social change 115
social construct 8
social context 15

social control 8, 80
social deprivation 159
social determinants of workplace health
    9
social divisions 9
social environment 35
social isolation 117, 120
social medicine 45
social origins of illness 40
social position 110
social relations 5, 113, 120
social solidarity 79
social structure 15, 40
social support 19
socialisation 76
socialised medicine 42
socio-technical systems 93
sociological analysis 12
Sorensen, G. 153
Southwood-Smith 29
Spain 22
Springett, J. 149, 164
Stalker, G. 93
Stamler, J. 22
Staples C.L. 12
Sterling, P. 77
Sterner, J. 77
Stogdill, R.M. 2
stress 6, 9, 12
styles of leadership 3
suicide 80
Sutherland, I. 33
Sutherland, V.J. 21
Svensson, L. 144
Sweden 96, 135
Syme, S.L. 22, 114

Tabor, M. 24
Taplin, I.M. 103
Taylor, F.W. 4, 18, 84
Taylorism 85
technological determinism 132
technology 3, 23
Teleky, L. 41
Tennan, H. 125
tension 5
Terryberry, S. 15
textile industry 38
Thackrah, C.T. 28
The Employment Medical Advisory
    Service 47
the historico-political approach 107

the nature of work 169
Theorell, T. 9, 10, 17, 19
Theson 45
Thom 45
Thompson, P. 110
Tory government 69
total workload 126
trade unionism 10, 27
Trahair, R.C.S. 96
Trice, H.M. 3, 95, 96, 100
Trilio Simpson Role ambiguity 21
Trilio, P. 21
Trist, E. 93
TUC 43
Turner, B.A. 96, 98
Tyrer, F.H. 47

UK 59
understimulation 124
University of Staffordshire and IRS 1997
    164
unwinding 126
US 59

Veterans Cooperative Administration
    147
victim 159
Viola, P.L. 44, 77
Virchow, R. 32, 116
Volpert, W. 19
von Bertalanffy, L. 93
Vuori's 138

Waitzkin, H. 37, 114
Waldron, H.A. 52
Walker, C.R. 93
Walsh, D.C. 153
Walters, D.R. 44, 45
Walton, R. 99
Wardell, W.I. 22
Warner 96
Warhurst, C. 110
Waterman, R.H. 98
Watkins 52
Webb et al. 78
Weber 75
Wedderburn, D. 78
Weindling, P. 40
Weiss, R. 75
well being 4, 9
wellness–illness dichotomy 1
Westgaard, R.H. 11

Westlander, G. 18
Wheen, F. 36
White, V. 144
WHO 7, 8, 69, 169
WHO WHP ethos 168, 170
WHP in Europe 165
Whyte, W.F. 96
Wilkinson, C. 143, 148, 150–151, 165
Williams, J.L. 129
Williams, S. 10, 144
Willis, E. 11
Winefield, H.R. 21
Wolf, S. 17
Wolinksy, F.D. 7, 8
Womack, J.P. 102
women 34; bodies 39; working lives 127
Wood, S. 103
Woodward, J. 93

work 74; health movement 32; hours 13; reform 141; stress 13
work/leisure relationship 126
workers 2, 16; alienation 77; participation 136
working class 34, 115
working conditions 6, 53; hours 20
working men's disease 38
workload 13
workplace 5–6, 108; health 25; health development 155; health promotion (WHP) 143; health promotion in Britain 149
Wynne, R. 143–144, 150, 164, 169

Zadjow, G. 9
Zaleznik, A. 12
Zeitlin, J. 102
Zohman, B.L. 13